WHEN
A CHILD
HAS
DIABETES

4th
Edition

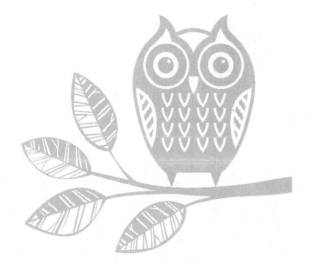

WHEN A CHILD HAS DIABETES

4th Edition

Denis Daneman, MBBCh, FRCPC
Shaun Barrett, RN, MN, CDE
Jennifer Harrington, MD, PhD, FRACP

The Hospital for Sick Children

Robert
ROSE

For complete cataloguing information, see page 232.

Design and Production: Daniella Zanchetta/PageWave Graphics Inc.
Editor: Sue Sumeraj
Copy editor: Linda Pruessen
Proofreader: Kelly Jones
Indexer: Gillian Watts

Cover image: Kids lineup portrait © iStock.com / FatCamera
Back cover image: Kids running © Squaredpixels / iStock / Getty Images Plus
Illustration: Owl © iStock.com / John Woodcock

The publisher gratefully acknowledges the financial support of our publishing program by the Government of Canada through the Canada Book Fund.

Canadä

Published by Robert Rose Inc.
120 Eglinton Avenue East, Suite 800, Toronto, Ontario, Canada M4P 1E2
Tel: (416) 322-6552 Fax: (416) 322-6936
www.robertrose.ca

Printed and bound in Canada

1 2 3 4 5 6 7 8 9 MI 26 25 24 23 22 21 20 19 18

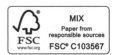

Contents

Acknowledgments

For those whose lives are touched by diabetes.
And those with diabetes whose lives have touched us.

We would like to acknowledge a number of individuals who have made direct and important contributions to this book. First, we recognize Marcia Frank, RN, MHSc, CDE, and Kusiel Perlman, MD, FRCPC, who coedited the first three editions of *When a Child Has Diabetes*. Both have since retired, but their impact on this book and on diabetes care within our team remains substantial.

Alison Campbell, RD, CDE, a dietitian on our team, made major contributions to chapter 7 for this edition. Other members of the diabetes team at The Hospital for Sick Children have given ongoing support and have reviewed the content along the way to ensure accuracy and comprehensiveness. They include our diabetes nursing and dietitian colleagues: Ana Artiles-Sisk, RN, CDE; Janet Ruston, RN, CDE; Catherine Pastor, RN, MN; Christabelle Almeida, RN, MSc, CDE; Lynne Cormack, RN, CDE; Esther Assor, RD; Vanita Pais, RD, CDE; Margo Small, MSW; and Ruth Slater, PhD, psychologist; as well as our fellow pediatric endocrinologists Drs. Diane Wherrett, Etienne Sochett, Jill Hamilton, Farid Mahmud, Jonathan Wasserman, Rayzel Shulman, Mark Palmert and Jacqueline Curtis.

We all owe a large debt of gratitude to Dr. Robert Ehrlich, the originator of the interdisciplinary diabetes team at The Hospital for Sick Children. His legacy remains firmly stamped on our team.

The book is written within the context of our diabetes service at The Hospital for Sick Children (SickKids), Toronto, and strives to meet the SickKids vision: *Healthier Children. A Better World.*

Foreword

The discovery of insulin by Frederick Banting and Charles Best, at the University of Toronto in 1921, suddenly and dramatically changed the outlook for people with type 1 diabetes. No longer was it a fatal disease, and no longer did health care professionals need to watch helplessly as children succumbed. Now there was treatment. The Hospital for Sick Children in Toronto quickly made a commitment to the care of children and adolescents with diabetes, a tradition that continues today. One of the first physicians to become involved in both diabetes care and research was Dr. Laurie Chute, followed by such eminent pediatricians as Dr. Harry Bain and Dr. Robert Ehrlich.

In the 1960s it became evident that diabetes care and education were too complex to be handled in the traditional medical model — that is, through occasional visits to the doctor by the child or teen and their family. Rather, what was needed was an interdisciplinary health care team consisting of physicians, nurses, dietitians and behavioral specialists, all bringing their unique training and expertise to bear on the care of this complex condition. The diabetes team was the first of the interdisciplinary teams now standard in many areas of health care.

Since most diabetes care occurs in the home, at school or elsewhere outside the hospital or doctor's office, care of children and teens with diabetes requires a family-centered approach: both the child or teen and the family are intimately involved in decisions that affect not only the diabetes but all aspects of their lives. It is essential that those affected know as much as possible about the condition. While we do not intend to present the last word on every subject, we hope you will find this a useful first step in learning about diabetes and its management, and a comforting reference when things seem not to be going quite according to plan.

Where does our information come from? We have all learned from our training, our mentors, our day-to-day work and, most particularly, from the children, teens and families whose experiences with diabetes constantly yield new information, new approaches and new coping strategies. Members of our team continue to be directly involved in the development of local, national and international guidelines for the care of children with diabetes.

We present this work in the proud tradition of excellence in diabetes care, education and research that has been the trademark of The Hospital for Sick Children for almost 100 years. If in some small way it lessens the burden of diabetes management for our readers, we will have fulfilled our mission.

Denis Daneman, OC, MBBCh, DSc(Med), FRCPC
Shaun Barrett, RN, MN, CDE
Jennifer Harrington, MD, PhD, FRACP

Introduction

Diabetes at any age can be a real challenge. However, learning about this condition, and how to manage or control it, is essential so that children and teens can get on with their lives with as little risk and as much vigor as possible.

This book is a practical guide for families of young people with diabetes and everyone who cares about them: friends and relatives, health care professionals, teachers, coaches, school bus drivers and camp counselors. In the majority of this book, the focus is on the child or teen with type 1 diabetes. Type 2 diabetes is the focus of chapter 6. Throughout, we will address these and many other questions:

- What is diabetes?
- What is the cause of diabetes?
- What is involved in "managing" or "controlling" diabetes?
- How do growth and development affect diabetes and, conversely, how does diabetes impact growth and development?

The information and insights presented here will interest both those who are new to diabetes in young people and those who are experienced with it. Each phase of adapting to the condition and each stage of child and family development brings new questions, concerns and expectations related to diabetes management. Families and care providers will find this book an excellent resource, but it has its limitations. It cannot and should not replace the comprehensive education program and support provided to the child or teen and family, at the time of diagnosis and beyond, by a team of experienced health care professionals, known as the diabetes team (see pages 22–23).

There are a few important principles to remember as you read this book. First, different diabetes health care teams have different approaches to some or all of the aspects of diabetes care we deal with here. If you are confused by something we have written, or it conflicts with the approach of your health care providers, discuss it with them. Most often you will find that what we have provided is a variation, rather than a radically different approach.

Terminology

When referring to someone who has developed diabetes, health care professionals most frequently use phrases like "children and teens living with diabetes" or "children and teens with diabetes." We prefer not to use the term *diabetic*, which is somewhat stigmatizing and fails to recognize aspects of the individual other than the diabetes.

Second, this book was written in 1998, revised in 2002 and again in 2009, and rewritten now in 2018 — things change! We expect that biomedical research will continue to advance our understanding of many aspects of diabetes care in the foreseeable future. So expect an evolution in our thinking in years to come. Perhaps the biggest change since the last edition is in the book's format. In order to make the information more easily accessible to the reader, we have created various boxes that provide, in each chapter, key messages, "recipes" for performing routines or approaching different situations, and examples of our experiences, which we believe will support the day-to-day management of children with diabetes.

Third, not everything works for everybody. If something doesn't seem applicable to you or your child, discuss it with your team. Once you have a good understanding of the condition, work with your team to do some further experimentation. Try things out and see how successful they are. If they work well, tell us about them — we're always ready to learn.

Finally, at times having a child or teen living with diabetes seems overwhelming. The message we wish to send is far more optimistic and hopeful than that. Present-day therapy has gone a long way to improving outcomes for these individuals and their families. Furthermore, advances in research are being rapidly applied to further improve the quality of life of those with diabetes. We look forward to the day when a book like this may be unnecessary.

Did You Know?
Repetition for Reinforcement

You will notice a fair amount of repetition in this book. There are two main reasons for this: first, the key concepts warrant reinforcement, and, second, the basics of diabetes care (monitoring, preparedness, observation) are needed in all situations.

Diabetes Self-Management Education

Both the American Diabetes Association and Diabetes Canada recommend that children and teens with type 1 diabetes and their parents/caregivers (for those below 18 years of age) receive *culturally sensitive* and *developmentally appropriate* individualized diabetes self-management education and support according to national standards at diagnosis and routinely thereafter.

- **Cultural sensitivity** is being aware that cultural differences and similarities between people exist without assigning them a value — positive or negative, better or worse, right or wrong.

- **Developmentally appropriate** means you use knowledge about child development to create a program that is suitable for the age and stage of development of your group of children. At the same time, your program considers the needs of the individual child.

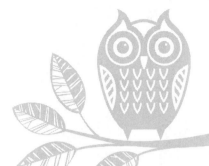

Chapter 1

What Is Diabetes Mellitus?

Diabetes mellitus is a group of conditions in which the body is unable to produce sufficient amounts of the hormone **insulin** from the **pancreas** to keep the blood **glucose** (sugar) levels within the normal range. The most common type of diabetes affecting young people is called type 1 diabetes. In this chapter, we address what causes diabetes, what happens when an individual develops diabetes, how diabetes is diagnosed, and the general principles of treatment.

Terminology

The phrase *children and teens* is used extensively throughout this book for two reasons: first, these are the individuals who with their families are the target of our book (that is, those under about 18 years of age); second, the use of both *children* and *teens* helps differentiate the younger children more dependent on family members for their diabetes care from the teens who are evolving toward adulthood and becoming increasingly responsible for their own diabetes care.

The term *adolescent* refers to the maturational stage from the onset of puberty to adulthood.

Key Messages

- Diabetes comprises a group of conditions that are serious, lifelong, and can have significant short- and long-term consequences/complications.

- Good (near normal) glucose control can significantly prevent or slow the long-term complications associated with diabetes.

- Health outcomes for people with type 1 diabetes have been steadily improving due to increasing research knowledge and better management tools.

Insulin, Blood Glucose and Energy

The human body needs a constant but varying supply of energy. The brain depends on a fixed rate of energy supply throughout the day and night. For the rest of the body, the demand for energy depends on how active a person is — less is required during rest (for example, sleep or time spent reading a book) and increasingly more during periods of light, moderate or heavy activity.

The Pancreas

The pancreas is an organ located in the abdomen, behind the stomach and nestled into the upper part of the small intestine. It plays an essential role in converting the food we eat into energy for the body's cells. The pancreas has two main functions. The first is the exocrine function that produces digestive juices important in the breakdown of the food we eat. The exocrine part of the pancreas comprises more than 95% of this organ, and it secretes its products, such as enzymes that break down food, directly into the small bowel. The remaining part of the pancreas, the scattered **islets of Langerhans**, is responsible for the endocrine function that regulates blood glucose levels. It secretes insulin as its major product, but also **glucagon**, somatostatin and pancreatic polypeptide. These substances are called hormones; hormones are secreted directly into the bloodstream and have their impact in other parts of the body.

Insulin is the prime anabolic ("building-up") hormone in energy balance. Insulin helps our bodies use glucose from the foods we eat to make energy. We need energy to help make our muscles move, our heart beat, our lungs breathe, our brain think — in other words, to do everything. That means we need insulin to survive.

Insulin is produced by the **beta cells** in the islets of Langerhans of the pancreas (see box). Insulin secretion is exquisitely regulated to keep blood glucose levels in a narrow "normal" range. The term "normal" here refers to people who do not have diabetes.

How Does Insulin Work with Food?

When we eat, the food goes to the stomach and the small intestines, where it is digested or broken down into components, or nutrients, small enough to be absorbed into the bloodstream and carried to every part of the body.

Food consists of three main nutrients: **carbohydrate**, protein and fat. Our bodies derive energy from all three. Through digestion, carbohydrates (such as those in bread, potatoes and fruit) are broken down into glucose; proteins (in foods such as meat and cheese) are converted into amino acids; and fats, including butter and oils, turn into fatty acids.

Glucose is an especially important source of energy, for two reasons — it can be converted quickly into energy when we need it, such as during work or sports; and the brain and nerves rely on a constant supply of glucose for their function.

> ## Did You Know?
> ### The "Insulin Key" Analogy
>
> Insulin is often described as a "key" because it unlocks the "door" to the body's cells, allowing glucose to enter and be used for the energy the cells need to function. In people with type 1 diabetes, glucose cannot move into the cells because there is not enough insulin in the body to "unlock" the cell doors. Therefore, glucose cannot provide energy to the cells, and it builds up in the bloodstream, resulting in high blood glucose symptoms.

In response to the glucose entering the bloodstream, the pancreas secretes insulin into the blood. Insulin stimulates the uptake of glucose by the cells of the body, so that they have the energy to do their work. Insulin also allows excess glucose to be stored in the liver, in the form of **glycogen**, or deposited in fat cells, where it becomes another important source of stored energy.

The insulin secreted by the pancreas in response to a meal is just the right amount to keep the blood glucose from going too high or too low. After most of the nutrients from the meal have been taken up by the cells and the blood glucose concentration once again approaches "fasting" levels, the pancreas secretes less insulin into the blood.

The Basal Amount

Our body is almost always producing a small amount of insulin, called a **basal** amount. This is needed because, between meals and while we sleep, the liver continues to release some of its stored glucose into the blood so that our brain and nerves receive the constant supply of glucose that they need to survive. This basal amount of insulin ensures that the balance between the amount of glucose being produced by the liver and that being used by the cells of the body is perfectly maintained to prevent either low or high glucose levels. Later, when we eat again, another burst of insulin is secreted from the pancreas into the blood, and the liver stops releasing stored glucose and begins to replenish its stores for later use.

Blood Glucose Levels in People with and without Diabetes

In summary, insulin is an essential hormone. It acts as a key, opening the door to the body's cells, allowing glucose to enter and to be used for the energy so vital to their function. Without enough insulin, glucose cannot be taken up and used by most of the body's cells.

In those without diabetes, the demand for and supply of energy are so tightly balanced that blood glucose levels remain in a very narrow range, and high and low blood glucoses (**hyperglycemia** and **hypoglycemia**, respectively) are prevented.

In comparison, in people with diabetes, there is a mismatch between blood glucose levels and insulin secretion or action, leading to hyperglycemia (high blood glucose levels).

Blood Glucose Levels in People without Diabetes

	mg/dL	mmol/L
Fasting	60–106	3.3–5.9
2 hours postprandial (after food)	<140	<7.8

Blood Glucose Levels in Diagnosing Diabetes

The following table provides criteria for the diagnoses of diabetes and prediabetes. Prediabetes can be defined as the in-between state when the glucose levels begin to rise but not sufficiently so for a diagnosis of diabetes to be made. It is, however, a high-risk state for later diabetes, particularly type 2.

Plasma Glucose Test	Normal	Prediabetes	Diabetes
Random	<200 mg/dL (11.1 mmol/L)	n/a	>200 mg/dL (11.1 mmol/L)
Fasting	<108 mg/dL (6.1 mmol/L)	108–126 mg/dL* (6.1–7.0 mmol/L)*	>126 mg/dL (7.0 mmol/L)
2 hours postprandial (after food)	<140 mg/dL (7.8 mmol/L)	140–200 mg/dL (7.8–11.1 mmol/L)	>200 mg/dL (11.1 mmol/L)

* Impaired fasting glucose (IFG) if fasting glucose is in this range.

The Different Types of Diabetes

The two main types of diabetes that can affect children are called **type 1** and **type 2 diabetes**. They have very different features (see table in chapter 6, page 90), and although type 1 diabetes is still the main type occurring in children and teens, type 2 diabetes is becoming increasingly common in younger and younger individuals.

Other specific types of diabetes include:

- **Gestational diabetes:** This occurs temporarily for a woman during pregnancy due to the hormonal changes associated with carrying a baby. It is often managed with diet and/or insulin.

- **Medication-induced diabetes:** This is a temporary type of diabetes that can occur when someone needs to take large doses of medication (for example, glucocorticoids such as prednisone) that, in turn, affect how the body's insulin works.

A history of other family members with type 1 diabetes is seen in less than 10% of families.

- **Monogenic and neonatal diabetes:** This relatively rare group of diabetes often runs in families, and is typically caused by a single genetic change. Children and adults with this type of diabetes can be diagnosed at a variety of different ages, including in infancy (often before 6 months of age). While insulin treatment may be needed for some, other types of monogenic diabetes can be treated with oral medicines or need no treatment at all.

- **Diabetes that results from a primary health condition or surgery** that affects how the pancreas is able to make insulin; for example, cystic fibrosis–related diabetes.

What Causes Type 1 Diabetes?

We do not know exactly why people develop type 1 diabetes, but research has given us some clues. Type 1 diabetes is classified as an **autoimmune disorder**, since the body attacks and destroys the insulin-producing cells (beta cells) in the pancreas. This is similar to other types of conditions, such as rheumatoid arthritis, lupus and multiple sclerosis, whereby the body starts to see a part of itself as "foreign" and the **immune system** responds by destroying certain cells. In type 1 diabetes, this autoimmune destruction eventually leads to very minimal and then no insulin production, which results in the body being unable to maintain normal blood glucose levels.

So far, researchers have identified two main factors behind this autoimmune response: genetics and environment. It seems as if both are needed for type 1 diabetes to develop: that is, genes that confer a high degree of risk for developing this condition, and an environmental trigger, or triggers, that convert this risk to disease.

Genetics

It appears that the likelihood to develop type 1 diabetes is inherited, but only some people born with a high chance of developing diabetes will actually develop this condition. In fact, a history of other family members with type 1 diabetes is seen in less than 10% of families. That genetic factors cannot be used to predict diabetes with 100% certainty suggests that other factors, likely environmental, may also be involved.

Environment

The exact environmental trigger or triggers responsible for diabetes have not yet been determined. Some researchers believe that certain viral infections, illnesses, or environmental or food toxins may either damage the pancreas directly or trigger the autoimmune response. Other researchers have suggested that an increase in weight or **body mass index (BMI)** accelerates the development of type 1 diabetes. Many children diagnosed with diabetes have recently recovered from a virus or other illness. But everyone gets viruses and very few get diabetes. Although high levels of stress or even the onset of puberty frequently occur around the development of diabetes, these factors are not believed to be the cause.

Signs and Symptoms: Type 1 Diabetes

- Urinating more than usual (**polyuria**)
- Getting up in the night to urinate (**nocturia**)
- Bed-wetting (**enuresis**)
- Thirst (**polydipsia**)
- Dry mouth, dry skin, sunken eyes — signs of dehydration caused by increased urination leading to fluid loss
- Weight loss and increased appetite (**polyphagia**) caused by loss of sugar in the urine
- Other symptoms: yeast infections, drowsiness, vomiting, fruity smell to breath (from **ketones**)

Note: These symptoms will also recur if the diabetes is not well controlled and glucose is running high.

What Causes Type 2 Diabetes?

Unlike type 1 diabetes, in type 2 diabetes the insulin continues to be produced, but the quantity and action are insufficient to maintain normal glucose levels. Type 2 diabetes occurs predominantly in the aging population, although younger and younger individuals are being diagnosed with this type of diabetes. In particular, individuals who are obese and/or come from certain ethnic groups (for example, Aboriginal Americans and Canadians, Hispanics, African-Americans, African-Canadians, Asians) are at greater risk. There is also a strong genetic susceptibility to type 2 diabetes. (See chapter 6 for more information about type 2 diabetes.)

The Stages of Type 1 Diabetes

Although there is much variability in the onset and course of type 1 diabetes, this condition often progresses through distinct stages. These stages are important when medical interventions are used to try to improve the early course of type 1 diabetes.

Onset

In people who are developing type 1 or type 2 diabetes, there will be minimal signs until the blood glucose begins to spill into the urine (called **glycosuria**) because the blood glucose levels have become too high and the kidney can no longer reabsorb the glucose (called the renal threshold). When this begins to happen, the water leaving the body takes the glucose with it, which causes excess urine production and more frequent urination (polyuria). This may be noted first at night if the child gets up frequently to urinate (nocturia), or if the previously trained child wets the bed (enuresis).

To make up for the loss of fluid in the urine, the child will become increasingly thirsty and drink more fluids (polydipsia). This is sometimes overlooked — for example, during hot weather. As well, a child's increased urination or frequency of having accidents overnight can also be attributed to them drinking more during the day and before bed. Eventually the increased drinking to try to compensate for the increased urination cannot maintain the fluid levels in the body and the individual starts to experience signs of dehydration, such as dry mouth, dry lips and sunken eyes. Over time, the presence of these symptoms should raise suspicion.

As well, since sugar is energy, its loss in the urine is often associated with fatigue, weight loss and an attempt to compensate by eating more (polyphagia).

In younger children, yeast infections (diaper rash or oral thrush) may occur. This might be easier to detect for children still in diapers. In teenage girls, yeast infections in the vaginal area may also occur more often.

In a child or teen with typical symptoms of diabetes (peeing more, drinking more), the diagnosis is confirmed by a random blood glucose level above 200 mg/dL (11.1 mmol/L). Differentiation between type 1 and type 2 diabetes is usually not difficult due to the very different populations each condition affects. However, when there is uncertainty, testing for **antibodies** to islet cell proteins, in order to determine any autoimmunity, is indicated. If these tests are positive for more than one antibody, the diagnosis is almost certainly type 1 diabetes.

Since sugar is energy, its loss in the urine is often associated with fatigue, weight loss and an attempt to compensate by eating more.

Pro Tip

In situations where a child is ill with no known cause, a family doctor should measure blood glucose levels or test for glucose in the urine.

Progression from Hyperglycemia to Diabetic Ketoacidosis

In type 1 diabetes, autoimmune destruction of the insulin cells in the pancreas results in not enough insulin being made in order to maintain normal control of blood glucose concentrations. As a result, even though blood glucose levels rise, in the absence of sufficient insulin, not enough energy can be provided to the cells of the body. The body then reverts to the use of fat as an energy source instead of glucose. This leads to the accumulation of ketone bodies as a result of excess fat breakdown. Ketones are acidic and can produce a life-threatening state called **diabetic ketoacidosis** (DKA). This state is less likely to occur in type 2 diabetes since some insulin is still being made.

DKA at Diabetes Onset: Key Messages

- When new-onset diabetes is diagnosed, treatment should be instituted immediately to prevent progression to DKA.

- DKA occurs in 15% to 30% of children and teens with new-onset diabetes.

- DKA can be prevented by testing for diabetes in any child or teen with undetermined acute illness.

Honeymoon Period

Once insulin treatment begins, the few remaining beta cells get a rest and actually start to better produce insulin for a limited amount of time. A few weeks after diagnosis, many parents are surprised to find that the insulin requirement decreases, giving the impression that the diabetes is going away. This is because once the insulin is injected, it cannot be turned on and off, as in the person without diabetes. This is known as the remission, or the honeymoon period. During this time, the pancreas seems to be able to secrete some insulin, but this is only temporary.

These changes in insulin dosage do not mean that the diabetes was misdiagnosed or that it has been cured. This period can last a few months or even a year or longer, but during that time, the pancreas continues to lose insulin-producing cells. As the honeymoon comes to an end, the blood glucose rises and the daily insulin dose should increase, usually gradually, to an amount more consistent with what a child of that particular height and weight would require. This increase in insulin requirement should be seen as part of the natural course of the condition, rather than a sign that the diabetes is suddenly getting worse.

> **Did You Know?**
> **Risk of Hypoglycemia**
>
> As the glucose levels decline during the honeymoon period, the individual with diabetes may be at risk for low blood glucose (hypoglycemia).

Settling in for the Long Term

Before thinking about the long term, children and teens with new-onset diabetes and their parents (or alternate caregivers) will need to figure out, with the assistance of their diabetes care team, how to live with diabetes on a daily basis. The expectation is that children and teens will be able to live healthy lives with type 1 diabetes, characterized by:

- An absence of high and low blood glucose symptoms
- Normal growth and physical development
- Normal school attendance and performance
- Plenty of energy for regular activities

Complications of Diabetes

Short-Term

- Uncontrolled high glucose levels associated with fat breakdown, which produces ketones, leads to diabetic ketoacidosis.

- Low glucose levels (hypoglycemia) can cause symptoms such as shakiness and tiredness. If not treated with sugar, severe hypoglycemia may develop, including slurred speech, confusion, convulsions and unconsciousness.

Long-Term

- Small blood vessel damage (microvascular disease) to the kidneys (diabetic **nephropathy**), eyes (diabetic **retinopathy**) and nerves (diabetic **neuropathy**)

- Large blood vessel damage (macrovascular disease) to the heart (heart attacks), brain (strokes) and peripheral blood vessels (poor circulation)

The A1c Test

Hemoglobin is the part of the red blood cell that carries oxygen from the lungs to the rest of the body. Scientists have discovered that in all people, whether they have diabetes or not, some glucose sticks to the hemoglobin and stays there for the life span of the red blood cell — about three to four months. The amount of glucose that sticks to the hemoglobin reflects the average blood glucose level during that period and can be measured in a laboratory using the **hemoglobin A1c test**. When the average blood glucose level has been high, the test result will be high. Thus, the A1c indicates the level of control over the previous few months. The level of A1c achieved over time is the best predictor of the risk of long-term diabetes-related complications such as eye, kidney or nerve damage.

What A1c Levels Mean in Terms of Average Blood Glucose Concentrations

A1c	mg/dL	mmol/L
5%	90	5.0
6%	115–125	6.5–7.0
7%	145–160	8.0–9.0
8%	170–200	9.5–11.0
9%	200–240	11.0–13.0
10%	230–270	12.5–15.0
11%	250–300	14.0–17.0
12%	280–350	15.5–19.0

A1c can be measured at any time, and often, enough blood can be collected for this test from a finger prick, although sometimes the blood sample has to be taken from a vein. There are different methods for measuring A1c. Some methods give immediate results; others take a little longer. Efforts are now underway to standardize A1c worldwide. In people without diabetes, A1c levels are generally in the range of about 4% to 6%. Nonetheless, you'll want to check the nondiabetic range for your laboratory. Even with intensive treatment, few children and teens with diabetes can achieve this level without risking frequent low blood glucose reactions. Instead, strive to achieve the best A1c levels possible. In the absence of many low blood glucose reactions, levels less than

Did You Know?
A1c: The Three-Month Test

Hemoglobin A1c is a measure of the average blood glucose level over the previous three months. This test is also known as glycosylated or glycated hemoglobin or glycohemoglobin. In our discussion, we simply refer to hemoglobin A1c checking as A1c.

Research Spotlight

Basis for the Current Treatment of Type 1 Diabetes

A landmark study was performed in the 1980–90s called the Diabetes Control and Complications Trial; its follow-up, the Epidemiology of Diabetes Interventions and Complications, is continuing indefinitely. These studies show unquestionably that achieving and maintaining better diabetes control, as seen by lower levels of A1c or glycated hemoglobin, is associated with a significantly lower risk of the onset and/or progression of long-term **micro-** and **macrovascular complications**.

Given the lifelong and serious nature of diabetes, it is no wonder that a diagnosis evokes a strong emotional response.

or equal to 7.5% are considered to be the **target range** for children and adolescents. Generally speaking, A1c levels between 7.5% and 10% suggest a need for problem-solving with the team and extra effort to improve control, and levels more than 10% are a worry and indicate a need for a concerted effort by child, family and team to avoid trouble.

Children should have their A1c measured every three months, and the results should be tracked to chart overall progress. Be sure to note when a different lab than the usual one processes the test — methods, and therefore results, can differ from lab to lab, giving an inaccurate picture of progress.

Reacting to a Diagnosis of Diabetes

The diagnosis of diabetes elicits many reactions in parents, children and teens. On learning that their child or teen has diabetes, most families will go through one or more of the so-called stages of grief, not all at the same pace or in the same way. Given the lifelong and serious nature of diabetes, it is no wonder that a diagnosis evokes a strong emotional response. Over time, families do adjust and get on with life as they knew it. They find themselves adapting and readapting to diabetes, and feeling some of these emotions again and again.

Grief is not neatly packaged in a certain sequence: rather, aspects of one or more of the five stages may occur at the same time. There is no typical response to the diagnosis of diabetes, and grieving is highly individual. Nor do all members of the same family respond in a similar manner.

The five stages of grief that have been identified are, in sequence:

1. **Denial:** They must have the wrong diagnosis. This cannot be happening to me/my child. I am sure it will go away soon.
2. **Anger:** They are wrong. Who is to blame for this?
3. **Bargaining:** If you take this diabetes away, I will…
4. **Depression:** I am too sad to do anything. This is a disaster. We will never be able to cope.
5. **Acceptance:** We can and will deal with this. This is what has happened; let's get on with this.

It would be unusual if the child or teen with new-onset diabetes and their family members did not experience at least some of these emotions. Research indicates that these responses are common in the first 6 to 12 months after diagnosis but settle down thereafter. The best way to address these emotions is to be open about them, discussing them with the health care team and other family members. Often the help of a mental health professional is sought if these emotions interfere with the diabetes or other aspects of the child's life. Ongoing problems with the emotional impact of the diabetes and/or early problems with management are important indicators of future problems. As many would say, "The best predictor of future behavior is past behavior."

Did You Know?
Depression

What we have learned from personal experience, but also from a number of excellent research studies, is that, following the diagnosis of diabetes, most children or teens and their parents express feelings of loss and sadness, and many feel isolated and friendless. Perhaps one-third have strong enough feelings to warrant a diagnosis of depression. Mothers tend to be more affected than fathers, especially in cases where the child is young, it is a single-parent home or when the financial situation is challenging. By 6 to 12 months after diagnosis, most, but not all, families have returned to their state of well-being before the diabetes was diagnosed.

The initial response to the diagnosis of diabetes will also be influenced by the family's prior experiences with the disorder. Do they have a family member who had difficulties with diabetes, such as short- and/or long-term complications? Are they worried that other members of the family are at higher risk for developing diabetes? The initial response will also be influenced by the family's usual responses to stress, and can also provide a window into how they might respond to future stresses, such as transitions from preschooler to school-age, or to adolescence and its many challenges, or to care in an adult facility.

There may be no way to prevent the initial responses to the diagnosis of diabetes, and, in fact, many of these emotional responses are part of a healthy adaptation to a new reality, this family's permanent life-change. We worry more when all family members are stoic — seemingly unmoved by this new diagnosis. The expression of emotion allows a family to move more quickly toward acceptance.

For more guidance on dealing with the diagnosis and adjusting to life with diabetes, see chapter 8.

The expression of emotion allows a family to move more quickly toward acceptance.

The Diabetes Team

To meet the complex and ever-changing demands of living with diabetes, all children, teens and their families should have access to and be able to work with an experienced diabetes health care team. There are a few essential things to know about the diabetes team:

Pro Tip

Never be afraid to ask questions. It's the only way to get the answers to the things that most concern you.

- The team should be **interdisciplinary**, with members drawn from different health care disciplines: physicians (either **pediatric endocrinologists** or **pediatricians** expert in diabetes care), diabetes nurses, dietitians (both often qualified as "diabetes educators"), mental health professionals (social workers, psychologists, child life specialists) and others. Each professional in this group brings unique experience and expertise to the care of the child or teen.
- The team needs to be **family-centered**, in that the child or teen with diabetes and their family are essential members of the team, and that decision-making includes them.

- The team's approach must be consistent and **evidence-based**, meaning that there is a **common philosophy of care** that is supported by best practice care guidelines.

Members of the "extended" team, in addition to other family members, include:

- Family practitioner or pediatrician
- School personnel
- Recreation workers
- Pharmacist
- Babysitters
- Others who share responsibility for child care

....

The child or teen with diabetes and their family are essential members of the team.

....

The Diabetes Team

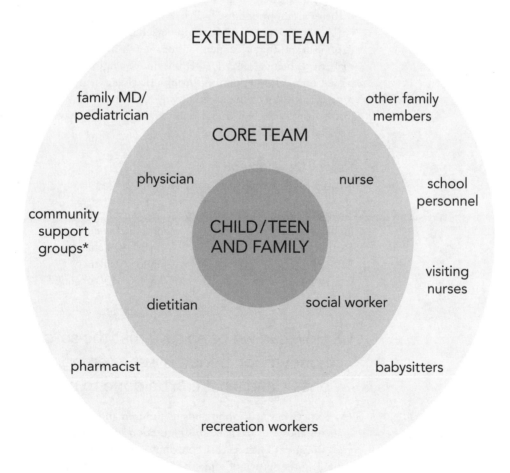

* Such as the American Diabetes Association, Diabetes Canada and the Juvenile Diabetes Research Foundation

Q & A

Q. Will my other children also get type 1 diabetes?

A. It's human nature to want to assign blame when something goes wrong. Many parents — and even children — are quick to take the blame for the diabetes. Women sometimes fear they didn't take good enough care of themselves while pregnant; some worry their child ate too many sweets or candies. But research shows that parents can't do anything to either cause or prevent type 1 diabetes. Nor can children. Children aren't born with type 1 diabetes, and at this stage, we cannot yet predict with certainty who is going to get the condition. Even if we could predict it, we would still have no way to prevent its onset. The table below shows the risk to other family members if one has type 1 diabetes.

While diabetes is an autoimmune condition, children with diabetes are no more susceptible to acute illness than any other child. Some people who have no personal experience with diabetes may be afraid that it's contagious or may think of a child with diabetes as being "sick." Diabetes is not contagious. It cannot be passed on to another person through sharing a drink, playing together, kissing or in any other way. Children with diabetes are just as healthy as their friends without it, once they have begun to manage the disease.

Risk of Developing Type 1 Diabetes if a Family Member Has It

Sibling (including fraternal twin)	1 in 20 chance
Identical twin	1 in 2–3 chance
Mother	1 in 50–100 chance
Father	1 in 16–20 chance
No family member	1 in 250–400 chance

Q. How can we be so sure that the so-called honeymoon period is just a temporary phase, and what can be done to prolong it?

A. Experience with thousands of children and teens with type 1 diabetes allows us to make this prediction with certainty. There are a number of factors that contribute to the honeymoon period, including the return of some insulin secretion from the few remaining cells that have been "overworked" by the high blood glucose levels. As the injected insulin brings the glucose levels down, these remaining cells recover and make insulin in response to the body's needs. In addition, bringing glucose levels down causes improvement in the action of the available insulin — that is, improved insulin sensitivity. Finally, appetite tends to settle down after a period of catchup for weight loss. However, as the few remaining insulin cells are destroyed by the immune process that causes diabetes, so the honeymoon comes to an end.

Q. My child asked if he was going to die because he has diabetes. What can I say to reassure him?

A. This is not an uncommon thought in young children, especially because the first syllable of the word *diabetes* is pronounced "die." The simplest answer to this question is a firm and reassuring "no" — no, they will not die because they have been diagnosed with diabetes. As a parent, it is important for you to understand that, in older people who have had type 1 diabetes since childhood, the long-term outcomes have been steadily improving and are close to the outcomes for people without diabetes.

Q. Sometimes I run into situations that I have never dealt with before and feel I need a little coaching. What should I do?

A. Your diabetes team is there to help with problem-solving. This means having access to your team when you need this help or reinforcement. Think of it as follows: Is the situation urgent or not?

Urgent Issues

- Illness with persistent high glucose levels with or without ketones
- Repeated vomiting
- Severe hypoglycemia

Non-Urgent Issues

- Planning for school trips or special sports events
- Questions about unusual foods
- Patterns of blood glucose levels that have not responded to the usual types of dose adjustment

If urgent, call a hotline number. Research an emergency service ahead of time, one that is open 24 hours a day, seven days a week. If not urgent, call one of the members of your diabetes team at a convenient time to discuss the problem.

Chapter 2

Supporting Diabetes Care at Home

This chapter deals with the specific tasks to be accomplished immediately after the diagnosis of type 1 diabetes has been made. Independent of whether your child or teen is admitted to the hospital at the time of diagnosis, your family will need to know how to give insulin injections and monitor blood glucose and urine/blood ketones. These are the first steps in learning about and directly managing diabetes. The details of recognizing and responding to patterns of blood glucose will be dealt with in chapter 3.

Parents quickly learn what they need to do to keep their child healthy and are able to follow through in performing blood glucose checks and administering insulin.

Key Messages

To ensure that your child or teen with new-onset type 1 diabetes is safe at home, your family will need to immediately acquire what are called survival skills, specifically the ability to:

- Monitor blood glucose
- Administer insulin injections
- Check urine or blood ketones
- Recognize and treat low blood glucose reactions (hypoglycemia)

Needing to learn and then follow through with these diabetes management skills at home can at first be very difficult and upsetting for parents, especially those of younger children, who often do not understand why these tasks are being done. However, in our experience, parents quickly learn what they need to do to keep their child healthy and are able to follow through in performing blood glucose checks and administering insulin. As well, children themselves are quite resilient and trust that their parents are not doing harm to them. Often just being in the home environment itself and carrying out these skills helps children be more cooperative, likely because they are in a familiar setting and have other normal routines occupying a larger part of their day.

In the early days following diagnosis, you will set up a structured schedule with your nurse and dietitian around the timing of meals and snacks throughout the day. Since food impacts the blood glucose levels, eating at consistent times is important to achieve accurate results and overall blood glucose balance. If your child already has a consistent routine, which is often the case with those in school, then hopefully there will be minimal changes to when meal and snack times are, and the diabetes care routines can fit into an existing schedule. (See chapters 7 and 10 for more information about the dietary management of type 1 diabetes.)

Blood Glucose Monitoring

Blood glucose monitoring is of critical importance in guiding treatment and in assessing the effectiveness of the treatment plan (regimen). Starting at diagnosis, blood glucose results provide the crucial information to guide insulin dose adjustments promptly and safely. Beyond the initial stabilization phase, blood glucose monitoring is essential to targeting and maintaining good glucose control and responding to unusual situations, including changing exercise patterns, food intake or an intercurrent illness.

When to Monitor

Blood glucose levels should be checked *at least* four times a day:

1. Before breakfast
2. Before lunch
3. Before dinner
4. Before bedtime

Blood glucose checks 90 to 120 minutes after a meal may be recommended to provide information about how well the insulin is matching the mealtime carbohydrate content and whether the pre-meal dose of fast-acting insulin is working well enough.

Pro Tip

There is good evidence that the more tests that are performed, the better the blood glucose achieved.

Your family will need to work out, with the help of your diabetes team, how best to do blood glucose checks (and possibly insulin injections) at lunchtime during school. The involvement of school personnel in this, most especially in supporting younger children, will vary from family to family and may also involve visiting nursing services.

How to Monitor

Since about 1980 it has been possible for people with diabetes to check their blood glucose levels themselves with a blood glucose meter. These meters require that a drop of blood from a finger prick be applied to a strip in a glucose meter. The accuracy of these meters/strips has dramatically improved over time.

There are many good monitors available, and over time you may switch to a different meter that has features that suit your child or teen best. Regardless of what monitor your child has, the best one is one that is used often, with results frequently looked at to make treatment decisions. (See chapter 3 for more information about blood glucose measurement devices, including continuous blood glucose sensors, and tracking blood glucose to make dose changes.)

> Regardless of what monitor your child has, the best one is one that is used often, with results frequently looked at to make treatment decisions.

HOW TO: Do a Blood Glucose Check

To test the blood glucose level, you will need a blood glucose meter and a testing kit that includes a lancing device (also called a finger poker), lancets and test strips.

1. Wash and dry your hands.
2. Insert a test strip into the blood glucose meter.
3. Prepare the lancing device by removing the cap and inserting a lancet. Twist off and remove the lancet cover, then replace the cap of the lancing device.
4. Pick a finger and push the button on the lancing device to give the finger a poke.
5. Gently squeeze the finger to get a drop of blood and apply blood to the test strip.
6. Record the blood glucose level reported by the meter in a logbook.
7. Change the lancet once a day, disposing of the lancet in a sharps container.

Checking for Ketones

When our body cannot use glucose for energy because of a lack of insulin, it turns to our fat and protein stores. As our bodies break down fats, they produce a toxic by-product called ketones, which can make children and teens with diabetes very unwell. Ketones are a type of acetone that can be checked for in urine or blood.

Pro Tip

At the time of diagnosis, or when your child is unwell with an intercurrent illness, urine or blood ketones should be checked until they are negative. This provides a measure of safety.

Testing for Ketones in the Urine

1. Take one test strip out of the Ketostix container and recap the container carefully.

2. Briefly dip the test strip in the urine, or wet the test strip in the urine stream.

3. After 15 seconds, compare the color on the test strip to those on the container label. Do not read beyond the 15 seconds.

4. Record the result of ketones and the time of testing.

Checking Blood Ketones

Blood ketone checks may be particularly useful for young children who are unable to provide a urine specimen on demand. A special meter capable of measuring blood ketones is required for this purpose. As well, different strips for testing ketones will be necessary, and often a larger sample of blood will be needed than is the case with blood glucose checks. Steps to check blood ketones are exactly the same as those used for a blood glucose check.

Pro Tip

Ketone test strips expire six months after the container is opened.

Understanding What Blood Ketone Results Mean	
Ketone	Blood Ketone Result
Negative	<0.6 mmol/L
Small	0.6–1.5 mmol/L
Moderate	1.5–3.0 mmol/L
Large–Very Large	>3.0 mmol/L

Preparing and Administering Insulin Injections

Often, for parents of children who have been newly diagnosed, injecting their child with insulin is the biggest hurdle to overcome. Many are squeamish about needles, never mind giving one to their own child. Teenagers, and indeed some younger children, quickly become quite skilled at administering their own insulin. Initially, however, all caregivers need to become good at this too. Other people closely involved in your child's life, such as grandparents, family friends and babysitters, should also be able to give an injection in case of illness or emergency.

Children who are preparing and injecting their own insulin must be supervised very closely at first to ensure:

- The *right type and amount* of insulin is being given *at the right time.*
- The full dosage of insulin is being properly administered.
- All appropriate injection sites are being used.

Teenagers, and indeed some younger children, quickly become quite skilled at administering their own insulin.

Using Insulin Pen Devices

Although syringes are still used by some people with diabetes to administer insulin, the majority are using insulin pen devices, which are a much more convenient and easier way to learn how to give insulin. Rather than withdrawing insulin from a bottle, you use a cartridge of insulin that fits into a pen-like device that has a special needle tip that screws onto the end of the pen. By turning the dial on the side of the pen, you can set the dose. When you push down on the end of the pen (like a plunger), the insulin is delivered. Each 3-mL cartridge holds 300 units of insulin. Some insulin pens are able to measure doses in half-unit increments, a feature that is important for young children requiring smaller doses. Needles of a shorter length can also be used with insulin pen devices, which often makes them less intimidating to children and teens.

For instructions on preparing the pen device to administer an insulin dose and on giving an insulin injection using a pen device, see Further Resources, "Using an Insulin Pen." But remember, these are skills that you should first perform with a member of your child's diabetes team.

Pro Tip

Many insulin pen devices are reusable, but there are also disposable pens available that come with the insulin cartridge already loaded in the pen device.

Diabetes Identification

All children and teens with diabetes should have readily accessible identification at all times in case of an urgent need for assistance from someone unaware of their medical history. The most frequently used identification is a medical-alert bracelet or necklace that states the presence of type 1 diabetes and includes the name and number of someone to contact for further medical or personal information.

The U.S. MedicAlert Foundation can be accessed at www.medicalert.org; the Canadian MedicAlert Foundation can be accessed at www.medicalert.ca.

Both foundations offer programs to support the costs of these products, which include enrollment and monthly fee, plus the initial costs of the products.

Rotating Injection Sites

There are four main places (sites) where insulin can be given: the arms, the buttocks, the abdomen or the thighs. In the beginning, you should try using a different injection area each time. This will help your child become comfortable with different sites. Ensure that each injection is about 1 inch (2.5 cm) or two finger widths from the previous one.

Many people with diabetes — and especially children — develop "favorite" injection sites, where the pain seems to be less and injections seem easier. If the same small area is used repeatedly, the fat tissue below the skin swells (**lipo-hypertrophy**). This creates large bumps that may lead to poor insulin absorption, which can lead to poor diabetes control. They may go away in time when the injection site is left alone. Until the bumps have disappeared, inject into another area to promote better insulin absorption.

At each clinic visit, a member of the diabetes team will examine the injection sites to help with site selection and the prevention of lumps and bumps.

> In the beginning, try using a different injection area each time.

Recognizing and Treating Hypoglycemia

For someone with type 1 diabetes, once the dose of insulin has been given into the fat tissue, the body cannot "turn off" how the insulin works, unlike individuals who don't have diabetes and are able to switch on and switch off insulin production as needed. As a result, if there isn't enough food intake to balance the insulin dose, or if there is an added demand for glucose during, say, intense exercise, the blood glucose may decrease below 72 mg/dL (4 mmol/L), causing low blood glucose symptoms, called hypoglycemia.

Did You Know?
Acting on Hypoglycemia

Hypoglycemia is rare in the immediate period after diagnosis, but action should be taken if signs of low blood glucose are present: check the glucose level and eat or drink about half an ounce (15 grams) of carbohydrate (for example, half a cup of fruit juice or two to three glucose tablets) and recheck the glucose in 15 minutes to be sure it is no longer low.

The individual signs and treatment of hypoglycemia are dealt with in greater detail in chapter 5. However, in brief, the symptoms of hypoglycemia generally fit into two categories: mild hypoglycemia results in autonomic symptoms (symptoms that are activated by the nervous system); moderate hypoglycemia results in neuroglycopenic symptoms due to a lack of glucose in the brain. Both types of symptoms can be limited by frequent blood glucose monitoring to identify impending lows and by eating appropriately and planning for extra exercise.

Signs and Symptoms: Hypoglycemia

Autonomic Symptoms

- Shakiness — "butterflies," feeling nervous for no reason
- Pounding heart
- Cold, clammy sweatiness

- Dilated pupils, "funny-looking" eyes
- Hunger, and sometimes nausea due to the hunger
- Change in skin color, paleness in the face

Neuroglycopenic Symptoms

- Lack of energy — tired, weak, floppy
- Lack of concentration
- Mood change — for example, irritable, grouchy, impatient

- Blurred vision
- Poor sleep patterns — restlessness, crying out, sleepwalking or nightmares

Q & A

Q. My child is struggling with doing his blood glucose check at lunch. Can we skip doing this during the weekdays while he's at school?

A. There are many factors that can change blood glucose levels on a daily basis, and this information is needed to make insulin dose changes. As a result, doing at least four blood glucose checks each day is essential, beginning right when you first learn this skill and continuing on an ongoing basis. Speak with your diabetes team about supports that can be put in place to help your child carry out this routine while he's at school.

Q. I hate needles. How can I expect my 6-year-old to get used to them?

A. Children take their cues from their parents. Any fear or dislike you have of needles may make your child afraid too. Some parents find that reminding themselves that the insulin injection allows their child to survive and stay healthy makes injection time easier. If parents say, "I need to give you your insulin so you'll have lots of energy to play and to grow," the child begins to understand, and the parents get over their own apprehension. Follow up each needle with a big hug and kiss, and get on with the day's activities.

> Even at younger ages, many children are curious and want to take part in some aspects of the injection routine.

Q. How old do children have to be before they can give their own injections?

A. There's no magic age at which children are suddenly capable. Generally, by 9 or 10 years of age, they have the manual dexterity and ability to give their own insulin. However, children this age may lack judgment. Thus, they usually require supervision into their teenage years. This means watching your child prepare the dose and insert the needle, checking the expiry date on the insulin bottle and reminding your child to rotate injection sites.

Even at younger ages, many children are curious and want to take part in some aspects of the injection routine. As they reach the age when they want to go on sleepovers or spend more time away from home, it will become more important for them to show that they can safely manage their own diabetes routines. This is a gradual process for both parents and child. Many children learn to give their first needle or to try new sites at diabetes summer camps.

Q. My teenage son doesn't like to wear his medical-alert bracelet. How can I convince him it's the right thing to do?

A. While some children feel self-conscious about labeling themselves as having a special condition, these little medallions can be lifesavers. Remind your son that the older he gets, the more time he will spend away from you, and with people who don't necessarily know he has diabetes. Explore sports-type medical-alert bands that he might be more open to wearing, or other options such as a medical-alert dog-tag necklace or metal wallet card.

Did You Know?
Icebreaker

Many young people find that wearing a medical-alert bracelet can be an icebreaker when they are unsure about raising the subject of diabetes. When new friends ask about the bracelet, they have the opportunity to explain, if they choose to do so.

Chapter 3

Striking a Balance

In this chapter, we address the factors that need to be considered to achieve and maintain good glucose control. To do this we need to describe how glucose balance is achieved in someone who does not have diabetes.

Key Messages

- Regular blood glucose checks are necessary to guide management decisions and to maintain the best possible blood glucose control.

- Keeping to a regular routine will help reduce the fluctuations in blood glucose levels and lead to better problem-solving when levels are outside of target range.

- It's hard work achieving consistent blood glucose balance, but it's well worth it!

When you eat, blood glucose levels go up. When you exercise, blood glucose levels often go down.

Blood glucose levels can change throughout the day. Think of a teeter-totter. When you eat, blood glucose levels go up. When you exercise, blood glucose levels often go down. In people without diabetes, the pancreas automatically changes the amount of insulin produced to keep blood glucose levels in the "normal" range. People with diabetes inject insulin in an attempt to mimic the body's natural insulin production as closely as possible. However, injected insulin cannot perfectly match the changes in blood glucose levels, so someone with diabetes has to work constantly to keep the teeter-totter from tipping too much from one side to another.

When there is a mismatch between food and insulin, the child or teen with diabetes runs the risk of high or low blood glucose levels.

- If there isn't enough glucose in the body to work with the insulin, they may experience low blood glucose, or hypoglycemia.
- If there is too much food for the given amount of insulin, they could have high blood glucose, or hyperglycemia.

The main goal of diabetes management is to restore and maintain blood glucose balance. At diagnosis, the first step is to reverse any symptoms of high blood glucose with the administration of insulin. Following this acute stage, the next step is to match the child's or teen's appetite and dietary needs for growth and development with the right amount of insulin. As children continue to grow and develop, their insulin needs change alongside their changing activities and lifestyles, and will need to be monitored on an ongoing basis.

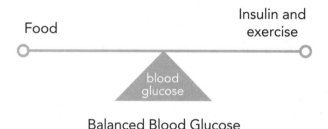

Balanced Blood Glucose

Did You Know?
Keep Learning

Knowledge is the cornerstone of managing diabetes. Learning as much as you can about diabetes and how to manage it will help you feel more secure and will decrease your fears and concerns. The goal of diabetes management is to help children live long, healthy, productive lives, as much as possible like any other child or teen.

CASE HISTORY
Taking Responsibility

Nicole has had diabetes for one year. At age 14, just a year after being diagnosed, Nicole has taken on many of the responsibilities for her diabetes care. She checks her blood glucose four times a day and gives her own insulin injections. She can feel when her blood glucose levels go low and is able to manage these episodes. While most of her blood glucose levels are in her target range of 70 to 145 mg/dL (4 to 8 mmol/L), she does still have some occasional higher readings, often after eating more snacks than she meant to after school.

Gaining Day-to-Day Blood Glucose Balance

Children with good diabetes control can be expected to enjoy general physical and emotional well-being.

Before thinking about the future, children with diabetes and their parents need to figure out how to live with diabetes from day to day. Children with good diabetes control can be expected to enjoy general physical and emotional well-being, characterized by:

- No symptoms of high blood glucose levels (for example, increased urination and thirst)
- Infrequent low blood glucose symptoms
- Normal growth and physical development
- Lots of energy
- Interest in friends and activities
- Regular school attendance and performance

Research Spotlight

Better Blood Glucose Control Means Better Health

Paying close attention to the blood glucose balance day after day is hard work. But over the long run, it's worth it. In 1993, the results of an important study, the Diabetes Control and Complications Trial, showed that good blood glucose control over time makes a difference to future health. The better the control, the less likely it is that long-term complications to eyes, kidneys, blood vessels and nerves will develop.

"Predictable" Factors That Affect Blood Glucose Balance

Insulin, foods containing carbohydrate, and activity are considered "predictable" factors that affect blood glucose balance, given that there is some element of control in influencing how these factors change specific blood glucose levels.

Insulin

In people without diabetes, the pancreas delivers tiny amounts of insulin all the time and secretes extra insulin when you eat in order to prevent increases in blood glucose. Injected insulin is administered in order to perform a similar function in those living with type 1 diabetes. There are several different insulin regimens. Deciding which works best for your child or teen depends on several factors, such as their age and daily routine.

Examples of insulin regimens include:

- Two or three injections of insulin are given each day (before breakfast, supper and bed).

- Multiple daily injections: long-acting insulin is given once or twice a day (often before bed), and short-acting insulin is given before each meal.

- Insulin pump therapy: a continuous insulin infusion is given underneath the skin.

We'll learn more about the different types of insulin in chapter 4.

Food

It's important for children and teens with diabetes to maintain a healthy level of blood glucose by matching their food intake with the appropriate amount of insulin. There are different ways to achieve this.

- Those taking two or three injections are generally required to be on a routine where they eat similar amounts of carbohydrate at about the same time each day.

- Children and teens on multiple daily injections with fast-acting insulin with meals or on an insulin pump learn how much insulin they need to take in order to balance the carbohydrate content of meals and snacks. More frequent injections may seem like a lot more work, but in the long run this can better match the food eaten with the insulin injected, which should lead to better blood glucose control.

Activity

In general, activity causes the muscles to use up their own stores of glucose and then draw more glucose from the blood. In people without diabetes, during exercise, the pancreas makes and secretes much less insulin and the liver produces more glucose for the body to use, so that the level of glucose in the blood remains steady. Activity in the presence of insulin

> **Did You Know?**
> **Meal Planning**
>
> Most parents agree that meal planning and getting the food/insulin balance right are the biggest challenges in managing diabetes. A dietitian will help you to create a meal plan for your child, keeping in mind daily routines, family habits and favorite foods. The goal is not to restrict food but to embrace healthy eating and to remain consistent enough to be able to determine insulin dosages. (See chapter 7 for more advanced direction on how diabetes is managed from a dietary perspective.)

lowers blood glucose levels, because when the body burns more energy, it uses more glucose.

In children with diabetes, the injected insulin is unable to "shut off." The muscles continue to use up the available glucose in the blood, and the liver cannot release its glucose reserves. This can result in the blood glucose level becoming lower. Sometimes the glucose level doesn't fall during the activity, but it may drop up to 6 to 12 — or even more — hours after the activity is over. This means that children doing strenuous activity in the late afternoon or evening may be susceptible to late-night low blood glucose levels.

While most activities lead to a decrease in blood glucose levels, some very stressful or competitive activities (such as ice hockey or running sprints) may increase the glucose levels, because the heavy stress of the game increases "stress" hormones that work against the insulin.

For people with diabetes, exercise offers extra benefits. It helps improve the action of insulin, so that less insulin may be needed to maintain the blood glucose level. For example, an active person requires less insulin than someone watching television, because activity brings blood glucoses down. Regular exercise also seems to make muscles and other tissues

When Blood Glucose Is Too Low or High

Low Blood Glucose (Hypoglycemia)

Low blood glucose is usually below 72 mg/dL (4 mmol/L). Symptoms include feeling:

- Shaky
- Hungry
- Tired
- Grouchy
- Pale
- Sweaty

If not treated with glucose, the child can develop more severe symptoms, which can include:

- Confusion
- Slurred speech
- Unsteadiness when walking
- Unconsciousness
- Seizures (convulsion)

High Blood Glucose (Hyperglycemia)

High blood glucose is usually above 200 mg/dL (11.1 mmol/L). Symptoms of hyperglycemia include:

- Feeling thirsty
- Needing to urinate more

If not treated, hyperglycemia with a lack of insulin can lead to:

- Breakdown of fats (called ketones)
- Vomiting
- Dehydration
- Diabetic ketoacidosis

more responsive to insulin, so the body requires less insulin to move glucose from the blood into the muscles. As well, regular exercise may help decrease the risk of diabetes complications.

A child's diabetes care routine should take into account the amount of exercise or activity he or she experiences on a daily basis. Parents, and eventually the child, will learn to adjust the routines for special activities. Checking the blood glucose regularly and making adjustments based on the results will help maintain the blood glucose balance during activity. (For more information, see chapter 10.)

"Unpredictable" Factors That Affect Blood Glucose Balance

In those with type 1 diabetes, certain situations (for example, times of stress, illness or growth) can affect blood glucose balance. These situations are considered "unpredictable," since their timing and duration is typically beyond our control and cannot be planned for.

Stress

Stress generally increases the blood glucose levels. Stress is the body's physical response to danger. Stress triggers a surge of power-boosting hormones, such as adrenaline and glucagon. These hormones, in turn, stimulate the release of glucose into the blood. Because children and teens with diabetes do not automatically make more insulin to deal with this, they can end up with a high blood glucose level. Stress can be emotional, caused by exams or peer pressure, for example, or it can be physical, accompanying fever and infection. Stress can also come in the form of excitement over seeing friends and family, or anticipating a special occasion. The bottom line is that sometimes stress makes the blood glucose go up temporarily. During a stressful event like an illness, parents and child will need to check blood glucose levels more frequently and take appropriate action.

Growth

As children grow, they will need larger amounts of insulin. This will be even more obvious during growth spurts such as puberty, when larger amounts of growth hormone are released. This normal change occurs even in children *without diabetes*; studies have shown that the pancreas releases larger

Did You Know?
Understanding Your Child

You do not need to make any special attempt to create a "stress-free" environment for your child with diabetes. However, understanding what may be worrying your child is important when it comes to communicating with your child and deciding how to better balance their blood glucose levels.

amounts of insulin during this time due to increased levels of growth hormone, which affects how well insulin is able to work in the body.

There are other hormones that also affect the blood glucose levels. These are called the counter-regulatory hormones because they work in opposite ways to the actions of insulin. They include:

- **Adrenaline:** released during periods of stress (for example, emotional distress, physical pain, intense activity)
- **Estrogen:** changes before and during menstruation
- **Glucagon:** released in response to low blood glucose

Illness

When children with diabetes become ill — for example, with a viral illness such as a cold or the flu — their blood glucose level often increases, and ketones may show in the urine or blood. Illness is a stress to the body, and stress creates a demand for more insulin. People without diabetes automatically make more insulin at such times. Children with diabetes do not. Therefore, on a sick day, the usual amount of insulin may not be enough, and monitoring may show high blood glucose levels, with or without ketones. At such times, you may need to increase the insulin dose, even though the appetite may be poor, to prevent DKA.

Although all illnesses in people with diabetes must be taken seriously, not all illnesses make the blood glucose go up. In fact, illnesses like diarrhea may be accompanied by low blood glucose levels. Careful monitoring of blood glucose levels and urinary or blood ketones will help determine the effect of each illness and the appropriate response. (See chapter 5 for more illness management guidelines.)

Monitoring Blood Glucose Levels Regularly

Since about 1980, it has been possible for people with diabetes to check their blood glucose levels at home. While home blood glucose monitoring may not be quite as precise as laboratory methods, it is certainly accurate enough for the daily management of diabetes. Home blood glucose monitoring is performed with a small, portable blood glucose meter. Meters require a drop of blood from a finger prick or, for some newer meters, from an alternate site such as the forearm or thigh.

Pro Tip

During periods of growth or stress, monitoring blood glucose levels for patterns is important in order to make dose changes and to help bring these readings back into target.

Illness is a stress to the body, and stress creates a demand for more insulin. Therefore, on a sick day, the usual amount of insulin may not be enough.

The blood sample is placed on a small area on a special test strip. A chemical in the strip reacts with the glucose in the drop of blood and a small electrical current is produced. The size of the current depends on the blood glucose level. The current level is then displayed on the screen of the meter as a blood glucose concentration. Blood glucose meters provide accurate, quick readings when used correctly.

Did You Know?
Lancing Devices

Lancing devices are spring-loaded tools that, at the touch of a button, activate a lancet to prick the finger to obtain a drop of blood. The actual lancet is a small plastic insert with a very short needle tip end. The tips come in different sizes, or gauges. The higher the gauge, the finer the point, which helps to get a blood sample less painfully. In addition, home lancing devices make it possible to adjust the depth of the finger prick, which further reduces the pain. Even young children may be able to take their own blood samples with adult supervision. To avoid spreading infections, your lancing device should not be shared.

Each blood glucose check gives a unique and important piece of information. However, one independent check cannot tell the whole story. Checking the blood glucose level several times each day is the best way to determine how well the child with diabetes is balancing predictable factors that affect blood glucose balance — such as insulin, food and activity — as well as to troubleshoot if other factors such as growth and stress may be affecting the balance. For children and teens receiving three to four insulin injections daily, checking blood glucose levels before each meal and before the bedtime snack gives an overall picture of how the insulin is working. These results can then guide insulin dose adjustments and corrections right when fast-acting insulin is being administered.

Blood glucose testing four times a day (before each meal and before the bedtime snack) is ideal but may be a challenge. For example, a lunchtime check in young children in daycare or school may be difficult, and the support and willingness of the staff will be needed. Older school-age children may also find lunchtime tests inconvenient, but they should be encouraged to do them. Parents and the rest of the diabetes team should work to help reduce the barriers to lunchtime checking.

Pro Tip

An occasional check in the middle of the night helps detect those at risk for late-night lows.

Other Times to Check Blood Glucose Levels

Sometimes blood glucose should be checked apart from the routine — for example, before, during or after a vigorous activity such as a dance class or football practice — to determine how that particular activity affects the child or teen, or during illness or other times of stress.

In addition, it may be recommended that, from time to time, blood glucose levels be checked 90 to 120 minutes after a meal. This provides information about how well the insulin is matching the mealtime carbohydrate content and whether the pre-meal dose of fast-acting insulin is working well enough. After-meal checking is often more regularly performed in children who wear insulin pumps or who are on an insulin routine in which they take fast-acting insulin before all of their meals.

Other situations requiring additional blood glucose monitoring include:

- When symptoms of low blood glucose (hypoglycemia) are present
- During an illness
- At other times prescribed by the diabetes team, or when you are trying to problem-solve or gather information about the impact of a certain food or activity

Blood Glucose Record-Keeping

The first step in spotting trends in glucose levels is to set up a logbook and complete it daily. Effective diabetes management is like putting the pieces of a puzzle together, and you can't complete the puzzle without all the pieces! Many pharmaceutical companies provide logbooks specially designed for diabetes management. As well, most blood glucose meters support the downloading of information to either a computer program or a smartphone app that will organize the blood glucose results in a logbook format and use different charts and graphs to identify patterns. Parents and children can also make their own logbook or may be provided with record sheets from their diabetes team.

Regardless of what type of logbook format you decide to use, the following things should be tracked:

1. The time and amount of each insulin injection.

2. The time and result of each blood glucose check.

3. The results of any urine and/or blood ketones checks.

4. Any unusual circumstances related to the diabetes (for example, a missed snack, an illness or strenuous activity).

5. Any low blood glucoses, including the time of day and, if possible, the cause.

Why all the effort? Keeping accurate daily records and reviewing this information regularly will help parents, the child and the team decide when changes are needed in the insulin dose and/or meal plan. Without a well-kept record, it is almost impossible to recognize patterns of blood glucose levels and to make appropriate adjustments in a timely way.

If your child or teen is recording their blood glucoses more independently and/or downloading these results to a computer program or phone app, remember to check these records regularly in order to stay informed and to make sure they are checking their blood glucose diligently and recording this information accurately. Record-keeping can be tedious, so don't be surprised if your child needs help from time to time. As well, building in a regular time to review blood glucose levels will support your child with their day-to-day management and help you to make dose adjustments at home.

> Without a well-kept record, it is almost impossible to recognize patterns of blood glucose levels and to make appropriate adjustments in a timely way.

Setting the Blood Glucose Target Range

The blood glucose targets change at various stages of growth and development. Target ranges are set based on the ability of the child and parents (or other caregivers) to understand diabetes, interpret signs and feelings of low blood glucose levels, and act on them. They are negotiated with the diabetes team, all of whom should have the same goals for a particular child or teen.

Your diabetes team will work with your family to determine a blood glucose range that fits your child's age and stage of development. Sometimes, no matter how hard the parents and child try to monitor meals and snacks, no matter how carefully they stick to insulin regimens or how

Blood Glucose Target Ranges	
Age	Children and teens under 18 years
A1c	≤7.5%
Fasting/preprandial blood glucose	72–145 mg/dL (4–8 mmol/L)
2-hour postprandial blood glucose	90–180 mg/dL (5–10 mmol/L)
Considerations	Caution is required to minimize severe or excessive hypoglycemia. Consider preprandial targets of 110–180 mg/dL (6–10 mmol/L), as well as higher A1c targets in children and adolescents who have had severe or excessive hypoglycemia or who have hypoglycemia unawareness.

active they may be, not every reading will fall into this range. In fact, in the beginning, very few may be in target. It is not unusual for parents or children to feel they have done something "wrong" or "bad" if levels are off target. But try to avoid looking at each blood glucose check as a report card; rather, see it as a piece of a road map that helps you make appropriate decisions about diabetes management.

Q & A

Q. Why doesn't exercise always help bring down high blood glucose?

A. In general, exercise does help lower the blood glucose level. Very intense exercise, however, can sometimes lead to a release of stored glucose, which, in turn, increases blood readings. Also, once the blood glucose is very high — for example, over 300 mg/dL (17 mmol/L) — don't count on exercise to bring it down. The only thing sure to bring it down is insulin. In someone with high blood glucose and not enough insulin, the glucose level just keeps building up. Don't exercise if you are ill and urine ketones are present.

Q. My daughter isn't very active. I'd like to get her involved in something physical, to avoid increasing her insulin. What can you suggest?

A. It's great that you want to encourage your daughter to get more involved in physical fitness, but remember, exercise is not therapy. If she preferred books to baseball before she had diabetes, there's no reason to expect her to suddenly change. Nevertheless, encourage her to participate in physical activities. Activity should be fun. You might start with family walks and go on to other social activities she likes, such as dancing, bicycling, swimming or tennis.

Children with diabetes should have the flu shot and all the other recommended immunizations.

Q. Should my child have a flu shot every year?

A. Children with diabetes do not get flu any more frequently or severely than their nondiabetic friends. However, when they do get sick, the diabetes may be affected, as discussed. Having a flu shot may prevent your child from missing a few days of school, and head off a period of upset in diabetes control. Children with diabetes should have the flu shot and all the other recommended immunizations.

Q. When my son's blood glucose is high, I send him outside to run around the block. He seems to resent the fact that his sister gets to continue her regular activities while his are disrupted. Is there any way to get around this problem?

A. While exercise does tend to counteract high blood glucose levels, exercise and activity should not be considered a tool of diabetes treatment. There are other approaches that might work just as well. Try sitting down with your son and coming up with alternatives. For instance, if this is happening at the same time every day, maybe you need to increase the insulin dose that would affect this glucose reading.

Q. My 15-year-old daughter's pre-dinner blood glucose checks are either high or missing most of the time. I suspect she's snacking on the way home from school. Any ideas about how to approach this?

A. You're wise not to demand explanations for why every test result is the way it is or to accuse your daughter of cheating. This is a sure way to get no blood glucose readings, or made-up results. On the other hand, it is risky to increase the insulin dose if you're not confident that the readings are accurate. It could be that the checks are done just a short while after your daughter has been snacking. Some parents deal with this situation by saying to their teen, "It seems your blood glucose checks are high before supper. Let's put our heads together to figure out what kinds of adjustments might be necessary." This gives you an opportunity to explore some of the factors that may be contributing to the high level, such as being hungry and eating more right after school or on the way home. Then the right kind of adjustments can be made.

It is risky to increase the insulin dose if you're not confident that the readings are accurate.

Chapter 4

All About Insulin

In this chapter, we focus on all aspects of insulin — its discovery, the different preparations available, the modes of injection or infusion, and how to adjust the dosage to achieve and maintain excellent glucose control.

Despite the long history of diabetes, no real headway was made in the understanding of its treatment until 1889.

Key Messages

- There are several different preparations and ways that insulin can be given. In choosing an insulin treatment program (often called the regimen) for you or your child or teen, it is important to consider the advantages and disadvantages of each, and which will best fit in with your child's or teen's lifestyle.

- Insulin requirements change over time, with growth, appetite, physical activity or illness. Doses need to be adjusted to provide the best possible blood glucose control.

- Most important in achieving optimal blood glucose control is consistency with schedules and ensuring that the insulin doses are matched to the amount of carbohydrate eaten.

Despite the long history of diabetes, no real headway was made in the understanding of its treatment until 1889. German physiologists Oskar Minkowski and Joseph von Mering learned, quite accidentally, that the pancreas was central to diabetes. In studying digestion in a laboratory dog, they removed the pancreas to see the effect. When the dog started urinating more often than usual, the doctors tested the urine for glucose. Indeed, the dog had diabetes.

As doctors inched closer to finding a treatment, young people with diabetes still didn't fare well. Most died within a year of diagnosis. In 1921, the breakthrough came when a young doctor at the University of Toronto, Frederick Banting, and his student, Charles Best, focused on the unknown hormone produced in the pancreas. Still working with dogs,

Banting isolated a substance from pancreatic cells and injected it into a diabetic dog. The success was not immediate, but eventually Banting and Best treated the dog with the islet extract, soon to be labeled "insulin."

The next real challenge was to treat a human with this new substance. The first human treated with insulin was Leonard Thompson, a 14-year-old boy dying of diabetes and confined to his bed. He was little more than paper-thin skin wrapped around a skeleton. The first injection of insulin had no effect. A biochemist, J.B. Collip, purified the canine insulin, and after 12 days of treatment, the boy began to look like himself again. Two years after their landmark discovery, Banting and Professor J.J.R. Macleod (in whose lab the experiments took place) were awarded the Nobel Prize in Physiology and Medicine. Banting subsequently shared his prize with Best, while Macleod recognized Collip's efforts.

Types of Insulin

Since 1983, biosynthetic human insulin has been produced in a laboratory by introducing a synthetic human gene into bacteria or yeast, which then produces insulin identical in structure and function to that created in the human pancreas. Through further modifications, manufacturers can prepare insulins with different action times (called **insulin analogs**).

Manufactured insulin is generally categorized into four groups: fast-acting, short-acting, intermediate-acting and long-acting. Insulin preparations are also described according to their course of action: **onset** is the time taken for the insulin to start working, **peak** describes the period when the insulin is working at its strongest, and **duration** describes the length of time before the effect of the dose wears off. Taken right before a meal, fast-acting insulin begins to work within 10 to 15 minutes and helps to control the rise in blood glucose immediately after eating. Long-acting insulin analogs such as Lantus and Levemir reduce the blood glucose levels throughout the day and overnight.

The day-to-day variation in insulin action is greatest with the intermediate-acting insulins, such as Humulin-N or Novolin NPH, and less so with the fast-acting and long-acting preparations. Dose effect will also vary according to the site of the injection, the volume of the dose, the amount of exercise being done and the activity pattern of the day. Variation is likely greater when legs and arms are used as injection sites, and less so with the buttocks and abdomen.

Insulin's Effect: How Soon, How Long

	Generic Names	Brand Names	Appearance	Onset	Peak	Duration*
Fast-acting	• Aspart • Glulisine • Lispro	• NovoRapid • Apidra • Humalog	Clear	10–15 minutes	1–2 hours	3–4 hours
Short-acting	• Human biosynthetic	• Regular	Clear	30–60 minutes	2–4 hours	4–6 hours
Intermediate-acting	• Isophane (NPH)	• Humulin-N • Novolin NPH	Cloudy	1–3 hours	5–8 hours	Up to 18 hours
Long-acting	• Detemir • Glargine	• Levemir • Lantus • Basaglar	Clear	90 minutes	Minimal peak	Up to 24 hours

* These times represent averages for each preparation and may vary from person to person, from one injection site to another and, to some extent, in the same person from day to day. Newer forms of insulin continue to be developed, and so the above list is not exhaustive.

Insulin Strength

Pro Tip

If you obtain insulin in a foreign country, make sure you know what type of insulin it is, as well as the strength of the preparation.

In North America, insulin is dispensed in a concentration of 100 units/1 mL. It's available in bottles to be used with syringes, in cartridges that are used with insulin pens, and with some brands of insulin pumps. Pen cartridges hold 3 mL, or 300 units. Each bottle of insulin holds 10 mL, or 1,000 units. Stronger preparations of some insulin types are also available (for example, 200 units/2 mL of Humalog U-200).

Storing Insulin

Insulin can be kept safely in the refrigerator until its expiry date. After opening, most insulin preparations can be stored at room temperature for a month. Levemir insulin can last up to six weeks at room temperature.

Insulin is a very stable substance that doesn't go bad easily. However, if it is allowed to freeze or get extremely hot, it can be damaged. If a clear insulin preparation becomes cloudy or straw-colored, or if it has solid particles floating in it, it should not be used. With cloudy insulin preparations, such as NPH, it is natural for the white substance to settle to the bottom of the bottle over a period of time. This should mix easily into the solution. Don't use cloudy insulin if particles or lumps are floating around after mixing, or if solid pieces stick to the bottom or side of the bottle. To be safe, if the insulin is exposed to an extreme temperature — below 32°F (0°C) or above 90°F (30°C) — discard the bottle.

Injecting Insulin

Often, for the parents of children who have been newly diagnosed, injecting their child with insulin is the first and biggest hurdle to overcome. Many are scared about needles, never mind giving one to their own child. Teenagers, and indeed some younger children, quickly become quite good at administering their own insulin. Initially, however, parents need to become skilled too. Other caregivers, such as grandparents and babysitters, should also be able to give an injection in case of illness or emergency.

Children who are preparing and injecting their own insulin must be supervised to ensure that the dose is accurate, the insulin is actually injected and the child doesn't favor the same injection site day after day. Supervision will remind them that insulin is important and potentially dangerous if too much is given at one time. When parents and other caregivers are involved, the support encourages better family adaptation to diabetes. (For how and where to inject insulin, see chapter 2.)

Insulin Dosages and Frequency

Initially, the diabetes team will determine the insulin type, dosage and frequency. This is the insulin regimen. It can take a few days to a few weeks of fine-tuning to figure out how much insulin is required. There are several different insulin regimens, each with potential advantages and disadvantages. Deciding on which insulin regimen works best for your child depends on several factors, such as their age and daily routine.

Examples of insulin regimens include:

- Two or three injections of insulin each day (before breakfast, supper and bed)
- Multiple daily injections — when a long-acting insulin is given once or twice a day and short-acting insulin is given before each meal
- Insulin pump therapy (continuous infusion of fast-acting insulin and fast-acting insulin **boluses** given to match blood glucose and/or food intake)

While some children may manage to maintain excellent blood glucose control on just two or three injections a day in the beginning, most require a more intensive approach once the honeymoon period is over.

The goal of insulin treatment is to mimic the pancreas in terms of insulin response. Ideally this means that a small amount of insulin is being supplied to the body all of the time (basal insulin) and extra insulin is given with food or in response to an expected rise in blood glucose, such as with food (bolus dose).

Twice a Day (BID) Insulin Routine

This regimen is used only in certain situations, as it can be challenging to achieve optimal blood glucose control. This routine may be considered for infants and young children who go to sleep close to dinnertime or for older children who are really struggling with taking their insulin.

This routine involves giving an injection of fast-acting insulin with a dose of long- or intermediate-acting insulin before both breakfast and dinner.

Three Times a Day (TID) Insulin Routine

This regimen is when insulin is given at three separate times of the day: before breakfast, dinner and bed.

- **Before breakfast:** Fast-acting insulin is given to cover the carbohydrate in the breakfast. An injection of intermediate-acting insulin is also given to cover the basal needs during the day as well as the carbohydrate eaten at lunch.

Insulin Delivery Regimens

Insulin Regimen	Potential Advantages	Potential Disadvantages
Two times a day (BID)	• Injections only 2 times a day • May be more appropriate for younger children who go to bed shortly after eating dinner	• Can be hard to achieve optimal blood glucose control, as it is more difficult to match the food (carbohydrate intake) with insulin doses
Three times a day (TID)	• No injection at lunchtime (e.g., while at school)	• Need to have consistent amounts and timing of meals and snacks
Multiple daily injections (MDI)	• More flexibility in terms of the timing and amount of carbohydrate eaten at main meals	• Requires a lunchtime insulin injection • Must know how to accurately count carbohydrate content in food • Need to reduce carbohydrate eaten at snacks (i.e., between main meals) or give insulin with medium-to-large snacks
Insulin pump	• Most closely mimics normal insulin secretion from the pancreas • Most flexibility with meals • Fewer injections (pump site changes once every 3 days)	• Need to be attached to the device all the time • Must know how to accurately count carbohydrate content in food • If the pump or pump site stops working, there can be a rapid increase in blood glucose levels and ketones. • Increased cost for pump supplies

- **Before dinner:** A fast-acting insulin dose is given to cover the carbohydrate eaten at dinner.

- **Before bed:** An intermediate- or long-acting insulin is given to cover the basal needs during the night.

This regimen may be used in younger children who are not able to have a lunchtime injection at school. In order to have stable blood glucose levels with this regimen, the timing of meals and snacks should be consistent.

Multiple Daily Injections (MDI)

MDI is a regimen that can allow more flexible timing of meals, but it requires the family and child or teen to be able to accurately count the carbohydrate content of their meals and give an injection at lunchtime and possibly at larger snack times.

This insulin regimen involves:

- Giving a long-acting insulin once or sometimes twice a day as the basal dose.

- Giving fast-acting insulin doses before each meal to cover the carbohydrate that is eaten and therefore regulate the blood glucose levels after the meals. To work out how much fast-acting insulin to give, family members are taught about **insulin-to-carbohydrate ratios** (see box, page 52).

This regimen mimics more closely than the TID and BID regimens how a normally functioning pancreas secretes insulin, in that there is a steady supply of basal insulin with several doses of the fast-acting insulin to cover the carbohydrate content of the meals.

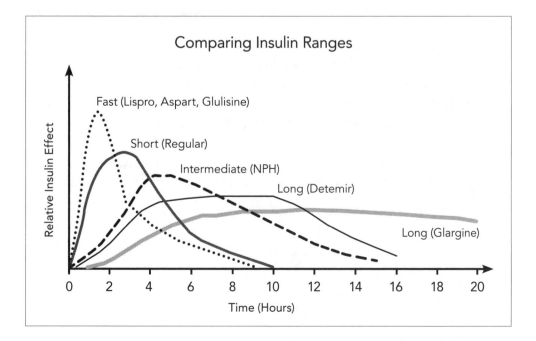

Comparing Insulin Ranges

Insulin-to-Carbohydrate Ratio

An insulin-to-carbohydrate ratio (I:C ratio) is the amount (in grams) of carbohydrate that 1 unit of fast-acting insulin will cover to keep the blood glucose level relatively stable. For example, an I:C ratio of 1:10 means that 1 unit of insulin will cover every 10 grams of carbohydrate eaten. A 1:20 ratio means that each unit of insulin will cover 20 grams of carbohydrate.

Calculating a meal or snack insulin dose becomes simple when you know your I:C ratio: simply divide your carbs by your ratio. If a child with a 1:10 ratio were to eat 30 grams of carbohydrate, they would therefore take 3 units of fast-acting insulin ($30 \div 10 = 3$).

The I:C ratio will vary from one person to the next, and may even vary in the same person from one time of the day to another. For example, a child might use an insulin-to-carbohydrate ratio of 1:8 at breakfast and 1:10 at other times of the day. Your diabetes team will help you and your child figure out the appropriate I:C ratio.

For more information about carbohydrate ratios, see chapter 7.

HOW TO: Make Injections Easier

There are many devices designed to make injections seem easier; however, none takes away the need for an injection itself. Before investing in any injection aid, talk to your health care team about its usefulness and effectiveness. If your child wants an injection aid to eliminate pain, remind them that all injections hurt a little. If the injection is more painful than usual, check the needle — there may be a defect.

- Insert the needle quickly — slow injections hurt more.
- Push the plunger in a little more slowly — this will reduce any burning sensation.
- Keep the insulin your child is using for that month out of the refrigerator — some children say they can feel cold insulin being injected.
- Pinch the skin less tightly or not at all if using very short needles.
- Try a different injection site.
- Avoid using alcohol to clean the injection site, or allow it to dry completely if you do.

If none of this works, talk to your diabetes nurse about the selection of injection sites, different kinds of needles and other tools that may be helpful.

Insulin Pumps

Continuous subcutaneous (beneath the skin) **insulin infusions** — otherwise known as insulin pumps, or CSII — are another way of giving insulin. When used correctly, an insulin pump, like the MDI regimen, more closely mimics a normally functioning pancreas than other regimens and allows a child to lead a more flexible lifestyle. The pump offers the potential for excellent blood glucose control with fewer occurrences of hypoglycemia, particularly overnight. It also allows for more flexibility in a child's food choices, exercise and sleeping. When a pump is used correctly, children are often able to achieve better blood glucose control than children using other systems of insulin delivery.

When a pump is used correctly, children are often able to achieve better blood glucose control than children using other systems of insulin delivery.

How Do Insulin Pumps Work?

The pump delivers a steady infusion of fast-acting insulin 24 hours a day. This basal insulin keeps the blood glucose level under control during times of the day and night when there is no food intake and protects the body from ketone production. However, basal insulin does not provide coverage for meals or snacks. The user has to program the pump to give insulin with food by pushing a button on the pump to deliver a bolus dose of fast-acting insulin just before food intake. The bolus dose can be adjusted for the person's glucose level, the carbohydrate content of the meal and the activity they are planning after the meal.

A pump is quite small and can be worn on a belt or on the arm, or carried in a pocket. The pump delivers insulin through a small plastic tube or cannula that is inserted under the skin, usually on the abdomen or the buttocks, and then taped in place. For some types of pumps, a length of fine, flexible tubing connects the cannula to the pump. For other pumps, the actual pump with the insulin is worn against the skin. The cannula stays in place for about three days. It is then removed and a new cannula is inserted at a new site.

Who Can Use an Insulin Pump?

Anybody with diabetes can potentially benefit from an insulin pump. Children are now starting to use the pump at younger ages, and sooner after diagnosis. In fact, even babies with diabetes can be treated with an insulin pump.

Perfect control of diabetes is not a requirement before using the pump. Many children make significant improvements in blood glucose control once they are using an insulin pump.

Pro Tip

Improved blood glucose control reduces the risk of complications down the road.

Success depends on both good family support and commitment on the part of the youngster with diabetes to make insulin pump therapy work. Good candidates for the insulin pump also:

- Come to clinic regularly
- Are comfortable with diabetes and willing to let others know that they have diabetes
- Are knowledgeable about diabetes
- Are confident in carbohydrate counting
- Are prepared to monitor blood glucose six to ten times a day, at least during the first weeks
- Have good attention to detail and good decision-making and problem-solving skills

If you think that you and your child can learn to use the pump successfully, speak to your diabetes team.

Advantages of Insulin Pumps

- For some individuals, it is easier to achieve good blood glucose control with a pump. You can adjust and manage insulin levels more precisely, with careful and frequent monitoring. Insulin pumps allow you to more closely mimic the normal action of a healthy pancreas.

- Pumps can help people achieve better long-term control as evidenced by a lower A1c — a measure of average blood glucose concentrations taken during the previous three months. Pumps may also reduce fluctuation between high and low blood glucose concentrations, and pump use is generally associated with a lower risk of hypoglycemia.

- The child needs only one needle poke about every three days to insert the new cannula. A push of a button delivers extra insulin when needed.

- The pump can be very liberating. Initially, learning to use the pump takes some time. However, subsequently, the child has much more freedom and flexibility to eat, sleep and exercise when they want.

Disadvantages of Insulin Pumps

- Because the pump delivers only fast-acting insulin, there are no long-acting insulin reserves to fall back on if there is a problem. This means that blood glucose and ketone levels can rise very quickly if something goes wrong with the pump or the pump insertion site. Blood glucose levels must be monitored more often.

Perfect control of diabetes is not a requirement before using the pump. Many children make significant improvements in blood glucose control once they are using an insulin pump.

- Some people find the pump is too noticeable — they don't want to be hooked up all the time and worry that it may get in the way of physical activity. Others find it is a constant, unwanted reminder that they have diabetes.
- Some children find that the needle hurts more, because it is a bit bigger than an ordinary insulin needle. On the other hand, there is only one injection every three days.
- The pump is only as good as the person who is running it. Anyone who is using the pump needs to be willing to make decisions and solve problems when they arise.

Concerns for Specific Age Groups

In young children, pump usage must be very carefully supervised by a parent or other responsible adult with knowledge of how to operate the pump and decide on insulin boluses. As the child matures, transfer of care will depend on their demonstrated ability to operate the pump effectively.

Babies and Toddlers

Babies and toddlers can be good candidates for the pump. Because they are with a parent or other caregiver at all times, that person can monitor the child easily and react quickly if there are any problems. Parents may worry that children of this age could accidentally push buttons on the pump. Most pumps, however, have a feature that allows parents to "lock out" the child so that only the parent or caregiver can administer bolus doses.

School-Age Children

Young school-age children often cannot count carbohydrates or remember to push the button on the pump before meals. But they are away from home during the day, so their parents can't be there to monitor the situation. In many countries, including most places in the United States, there are laws mandating schools to provide direct diabetes care (insulin injections, glucose monitoring). In Canada, there is highly variable support available at schools. Nonetheless, many families find ways to ensure that their children get the right kind of support during school hours. Discuss the possibilities with school personnel and members of your diabetes team. For some — for example, the youngest children — such support might mean that a nurse comes to the school at key intervals during the day to do testing and give insulin; for older children, support from a teacher or other school employee while the child performs the tasks may be all that is required.

It is important to
check blood glucose
regularly and address
any problems quickly.

Older Children and Teenagers

Preteens and teens are usually able to check their own blood
glucose concentrations, count carbohydrates and calculate
bolus doses. They can take on more of the routine of using
the pump. However, it's important for parents to stay involved.
One option is to sit down together at the end of the day to
review blood glucose readings and bolus doses. Parents and
teens can use this time to discuss any problems that came up
during the day and work on solving them.

Teens who are just starting the pump may be concerned
about gaining weight; if the pump improves glucose control,
this, in turn, will help their bodies use food more efficiently.
Weight gain is most likely to occur if blood glucose was poorly
controlled before initiating the pump. If this is a concern,
the teen should speak with members of the diabetes team in
advance and learn ways to minimize the weight gain.

Starting the Insulin Pump

Different teams start people on pumps in different ways.
All will ensure that you and your child have a training session
on the technical aspects of the pump. Many teams will use
this time to also update your diabetes knowledge and skills,
including carbohydrate counting.

Some programs — including ours at SickKids, Toronto —
recommend that children and teens wear the pump for a few
days with just saline (salt water) running through it. This allows
your family to get used to the pump itself; to solve any problems
with the tape, the catheter and the pump; and to go through a
set change on your own at home.

Next, you and your child or teen will come into the clinic
for the actual start. Based on information that you've gathered
through the use of food records and intensive monitoring,
members of the team will work with you to calculate and
program the correct basal rates. Similarly, bolus doses and
correction factors will be calculated and programmed so that
the pump is able to deliver the right amount of insulin to take
care of the carbohydrate in food and to correct blood glucose
levels that are outside of the target range. Your child or teen
will also be advised on how to compensate for exercise. You
will be asked to call your diabetes educator or doctor very
regularly, for a short while, to do any problem-solving that
is required.

As with any system of diabetes management, there is a lot
to learn at the beginning, but eventually it gets easier.

Potential Problems When Using the Insulin Pump

Because the pump provides only fast-acting insulin, blood glucose and ketones can rise very quickly if something goes wrong. It is important to check blood glucose regularly and address any problems quickly.

The pump is a mechanical device; therefore, it can break down. Problems can include:

- Batteries running low
- A mechanical problem with the pump
- A clog or a kink in the tubing
- The cannula slipping out of the insertion site
- Inflammation or infection at the insertion site, which makes it harder to absorb insulin

A pump has an alarm to alert the wearer when batteries are running low or the tube is clogged. The pump can be set to deliver maximum and minimum bolus rates.

If your child is using an insulin pump, you or your child should always carry:

- A blood glucose meter
- Blood glucose test strips
- Ketone test strips
- An insulin pen loaded with fast-acting insulin, in case of pump failure
- A supply of intermediate- or long-acting insulin if you are going to be somewhere where you will not be able to get a replacement pump within 6 to 12 hours if your pump malfunctions
- An extra set of batteries if your family is going to be away from home

Adjusting Insulin Doses to Achieve and Maintain Targets

Once we understand how the different types of insulin work and the various devices that can be used to administer insulin, a key step in achieving optimal diabetes control is to master the principles of insulin dose adjustment. A constant goal for diabetes care is to try to get as many blood glucose levels in the target range as possible, without too much hypoglycemia, so that the A1c can be as close to the goal as possible.

As children grow and their appetites and activity levels change, their need for insulin also changes. You shouldn't have to wait for an appointment with someone on the diabetes team to respond to these changes. Who better to monitor the changing patterns in your child's blood glucose levels and overall health than your family? Studies show that parents and children who actively participate in the diabetes management process are the most successful in adapting to this condition.

Remember that the need for more insulin, or even an increase in the number of injections each day, does not mean a child's diabetes is getting worse. Similarly, a decrease in the insulin doses doesn't mean the diabetes is going away. Adjusting insulin to the body's current demands is simply a way of maintaining good blood glucose balance and achieving better control. For example, a heavier child may need more insulin than a smaller child, and a child who is always on the go may need less insulin than a child who is not as active. A teenager will likely require more insulin during puberty than after the growth spurt is over. People generally need more insulin when they are sick than when they are well, and students may require more insulin during exam week, because of the increased stress.

To make independent insulin dose adjustments, whether they are temporary or permanent, families must:

- Be confident that blood glucose checks are accurate and meal plans are being followed (no secret snacking or skipping meals).
- Know the child's blood glucose target range.
- Understand the actions of the insulin types being used.
- Understand what each blood glucose check means (for example, after eating out or after exercise).
- Know when to contact the diabetes care team.

How to Think and Talk about Insulin Dose Adjustment

You will have lots of time to learn about and practice insulin dose adjustment with your diabetes educator. In the section that follows we'll give you some ways of talking about insulin and insulin dose changes. Having a common understanding of what we mean by terms such as *routine insulin dose* and *temporary dose adjustment* will help with our discussion on how to make these changes as needed at home.

Routine Insulin Dose Adjustment

This refers to a change in the dose of insulin based on a pattern of blood glucose levels taken over a number of days. The fast-acting, intermediate-acting or long-acting insulin may be adjusted as needed. Such adjustments are common in children especially at the beginning and end of the honeymoon, as the child grows or finishes growing, and when a change of season leads to altered levels of activity — for example, the arrival of spring, which has longer daylight hours.

Temporary Dose Adjustment

This refers to a temporary change in insulin dose to compensate for a temporary change in food or activity, or to deal with an illness. The fast-acting, intermediate-acting or long-acting insulin may be changed. It is assumed that the circumstances creating the need for the insulin dose adjustment are out of the ordinary and will go away, and that the insulin requirements will return to the routine dose.

CASE HISTORY
A Good Starting Point

Jane is a 10-year-old who has had diabetes for five years. She receives NPH and Humalog insulin before breakfast, Humalog at supper and NPH at bedtime. Jane's family has learned that each of the four daily blood checks is dependent on the action of one of the four insulin doses:

- The breakfast reading tells them how well the previous night's bedtime NPH (long-acting) is working.
- The lunch reading tells them if the breakfast Humalog insulin (fast-acting) is working.
- The supper reading reflects the action of the breakfast NPH.
- The bedtime reading tells them if the supper Humalog insulin is working.

These guidelines may seem a little simplistic, but they're a good starting point for Jane and her family when her blood checks are off target. When Jane woke up with high readings three mornings in a row, her parents knew she needed more NPH insulin at night. When she had a couple of nights when she was low before her bedtime snack, her parents decreased her Humalog dose at suppertime.

When to Make Adjustments to Injections

People with diabetes know when change is required by the way they feel and by the results of their blood glucose and urine ketone checks. Provided they are sticking to the meal plan reasonably well and/or using their insulin-to-carbohydrate ratio accurately, continuous high blood glucose readings usually mean that more insulin is required; repeated low readings usually mean that less insulin is needed. Generally speaking, you can assume that the insulin dose is right and no permanent change in the regular dose is necessary when:

- Your child or teen feels well and is free of symptoms of high or low blood glucose.
- The urine is free of ketones.
- At least 70% to 80% of the blood glucose checks are within the target range.

With any insulin regimen — be it two, three or four or more injections a day — it is important to know which insulin is acting when, and therefore which insulin dose needs to be changed when glucose levels are either too high or too low.

CASE HISTORY
Flexibility

Abdul is a 16-year-old 10th grade student and a competitive swimmer. He has had diabetes for eight months and has been on long-acting Lantus at bedtime and fast-acting NovoRapid before each meal. This routine allows him to have the flexibility he needs for his busy schedule. He checks his blood glucose at least four or five times a day. Each check gives him specific information about the effectiveness of a particular dose of insulin.

- *The pre-breakfast blood glucose result reflects the effectiveness of the long-acting Lantus.*
- *The lunchtime reading reflects the effectiveness of the breakfast-time NovoRapid.*
- *The suppertime check reflects the effectiveness of the lunchtime insulin.*
- *The bedtime check gives good information about how well the suppertime insulin worked.*

Adjustments
Using Pattern Management

Most people aim to keep blood glucose levels in the target range 70% to 80% of the time. Some variability is to be expected. The routine insulin dose should be changed only when a pattern or trend of blood glucose results are outside of the target range. If your child or teen is feeling well and has no ketones, it is time to make an insulin dose adjustment when the blood glucose is:

- High at the same time of day for three days in a row, or
- Low at the same time of day for two days in a row or three times in a week

If there is a good reason for the highs and lows, such as unexpected extra exercise or eating more carbohydrate than normal, the dose adjustment may be delayed a while longer, to see if the pattern persists.

How Much to Adjust the Insulin Dose

When the family has recognized that the routine insulin dose should be changed because there is a consistent pattern of either high or low blood glucose readings at one time of the day, we recommend changing the insulin dose by 10% (see box).

HOW TO: Calculate a 10% Dose Adjustment

To calculate 10% of an insulin dose, divide the dose by 10 and round down to the nearest whole number.

If the insulin dose is:	Adjust the insulin dose by:
Less than 20 units	1 unit
20–29 units	2 units
30–39 units	3 units
Over 40 units	4 units

Specific Guidelines
for Insulin Dose Adjustment

In the table on page 62 you will find guidelines for when and how to adjust the routine dose of insulin for patients on insulin injections. They go along with our diabetes education program at The Hospital for Sick Children in Toronto. If you are not part of this program, please discuss these guidelines with your doctor or diabetes nurse before using them.

These guidelines should be used only if your child or teen feels well and there are no ketones in the blood or urine. If ketones are present, more immediate action is required. Ketones should be checked when the blood glucose is more than 230 mg/dL (13 mmol/L) during illness. Information about how to manage blood glucose levels when your child is unwell can be found in chapter 5.

Once you have decided to change the insulin dose, it should be adjusted by 10%. For example, a morning dose of 20 NPH should be increased to 22. Once you have changed the dose, you need wait only two days to see if it works before changing it again. Once you arrive at a dose that gets the appropriate blood glucose into target, that becomes your new regular dose.

Insulin Dose Adjustments with Insulin Pumps

When diabetes is managed with the insulin pump, families need to learn how to adjust both basal insulin rate(s) and bolus doses. You may recall that the insulin pump delivers a tiny trickle of insulin constantly, day and night, and that this is called the basal insulin rate. Children who manage

When and How to Adjust the Routine Insulin Dose

Time of Day	If Blood Glucose Is...	Change to Insulin Dose	Which Insulin
Breakfast	Above target 3 days in a row	Increase by 10%	*BID or TID regimen:* dinner or bedtime intermediate- or long-acting insulin
	Below target 2 days in a row	Decrease by 10%	*MID regimen:* bedtime long-acting insulin
Lunch	Above target 3 days in a row	Increase by 10%	*All regimens:* breakfast short-acting insulin
	Below target 2 days in a row	Decrease by 10%	
Dinner	Above target 3 days in a row	Increase by 10%	*BID or TID regimen:* breakfast intermediate-acting insulin
	Below target 2 days in a row	Decrease by 10%	*MID regimen:* lunch short-acting insulin
Bedtime	Above target 3 days in a row	Increase by 10%	*All regimens:* dinner short-acting insulin
	Below target 2 days in a row	Decrease by 10%	

their diabetes with a pump give themselves extra insulin with meals or to correct a high blood glucose. This extra insulin is called the bolus dose, which is calculated to match the food intake (see "Insulin-to-Carbohydrate Ratio," page 52) and to correct blood glucose levels outside of the target range.

In addition to taking bolus insulin with food, people on pumps learn to take extra insulin when their blood glucose level is high and to reduce insulin when blood glucose is low. This means figuring out how much insulin is required to bring the blood glucose back into the target range during the next few hours. This is called the **correction factor** or **sensitivity factor**.

Families learn how to program the basic basal and bolus insulin information into the pump. By checking blood glucose results both before and two hours after meals, and recording or closely following the results online, it is possible (and important) for those on pumps to be on the lookout for patterns and to make overall changes in the routine insulin doses. When parents or teens discover a period of three days in a row where the levels are high at the same time of the day, or two days when they are low at the same time of the day, an insulin adjustment should be considered.

Adjustments Using Pattern Management

Similar to adjusting insulin on injection pump therapy, on an insulin pump, you will also be looking for patterns in blood glucose levels that fall *outside* your target range at the same time of the day. Remember that when adjusting insulin doses based on patterns, you are looking at *preventing* the problem blood glucose level rather than correcting it later.

Pattern Rules to Follow

- High blood glucose levels for three days in a row at the same time of the day
- Low blood glucose levels for two days in a row at the same time of the day

Adjusting Bolus Doses

- The bolus dose is calculated using the I:C ratio (see box, page 52).
- In order to be able to know how well the bolus doses are working, the pre-meal blood glucose level must be within the target range.
- The blood glucose levels that are obtained at two hours and four hours after a bolus tell how well the previous bolus worked.
- If the pre-meal blood glucose level is in target, the ideal rise in blood glucose two hours following a meal should be between 36 and 72 mg/dL (2 and 4 mmol/L).
- Increase or decrease the I:C ratio as needed by roughly 10% at a time:

Pro Tip

The longer the period between bolus doses the better when it comes to assessing basal rates.

I:C Ratio Adjustments	
I:C Ratio	Increase or Decrease to I:C Ratio
1:1–1:15	1 g carbohydrate
1:15–1:25	2 g carbohydrate
>1:25	3 g carbohydrate

Adjusting Basal Rates

- The blood glucose levels obtained more than four hours after a bolus usually tell how well the basal rate is working in the previous hours.

- Increase or decrease the basal rate as needed by roughly 10% at a time:

Basal Rate Adjustments	
Basal Rate	Increase or Decrease to Basal Rate
<0.3 units/hour	0.025 units/hour
0.3–0.5 units/hour	0.05 units/hour
0.5–2.0 units/hour	0.1 units/hour

Other Important Points

- The blood glucose result before breakfast indicates the effectiveness of the nighttime basal rate.

- Blood glucose results done two hours after correcting a high blood glucose indicate the effectiveness of the correction or sensitivity factor.

Adjusting Insulin and Food for Planned Activity

Most children welcome routines, but once in a while schedules change, and without adequate planning, the blood glucose balance may be upset. A weekly swimming lesson on Sunday morning, for example, will create different insulin demands than a weekly piano lesson on Monday afternoon. Parents and, in time, children can learn to assess the impact of these regular events, and when an opportunity for a new activity comes along, everyone will be better able to cope with the change.

Because exercise both lowers blood glucose and increases the speed of insulin absorption, it's a good idea to match it, whenever possible, with extra food or to reduce the insulin before the event. After a while you'll become more familiar with how your child responds to activity and you'll have a better idea of how much food, if any, to offer, or how much to decrease the insulin. For more information about adjusting food and insulin schedules for exercise, see chapter 10.

Q & A

Q. Our 5-year-old prefers that Mommy give the injections. Is that a problem?

A. In many families, one person takes on most of the responsibility for injections. Problems arise, however, when that person is unavailable. It's important that all regular caregivers are able to share responsibility for giving the injection, and that your child feels safe and confident with all of them. Single-parent families should enlist the help of a friend or relative. Some families work out a schedule where one parent takes care of the morning injections and the other parent looks after evening injections. Sharing the burden is also critical for coping with the daily demands of diabetes and preventing parent burnout.

It's important that all regular caregivers are able to share responsibility for giving the injection, and that your child feels safe and confident with all of them.

Q. What if some insulin leaks out of the injection site?

A. When insulin leaks, don't try to guess the amount lost and replace it. The risk of too much insulin causing a low blood glucose reaction outweighs any benefit. Note it in your logbook and take it into account if the next blood check is high. In the meantime, here are a few tips to minimize such occurrences:

- Get rid of any cause of excess pressure at the injection site, such as a bent leg or a chair pressing against the buttock.
- Inject the insulin slowly.
- If you are pinching at the injection site, try letting go of the pinched skin before removing the needle.
- Count slowly to at least five before removing the needle.
- Apply light pressure on the injection site for a couple of seconds as you remove the needle, to prevent blood and insulin from coming out.
- If you are using a short needle, discuss alternatives with your diabetes team.

Q. What does it mean if there is bruising at the injection site?

A. This can happen from time to time and it's not harmful. It usually means the needle has nicked a tiny blood vessel. To minimize the chance of bruising, apply gentle pressure to the site with a dry piece of cotton or a clean finger after injecting. Also be careful not to pinch the skin too tightly or insert the needle too slowly. If you get continuous and excessive bruising, consult your diabetes team.

Q. Why is the injection site all red and itchy?

A. Some children are sensitive to rubbing alcohol or one of the components of the insulin solution. The redness you see is probably hives — a localized allergic reaction. Changing the brand of insulin may help. In rare cases, someone has an allergic reaction to insulin. Speak to your diabetes team. In most cases, the child eventually builds up a tolerance to the insulin and the reaction subsides.

Q. What happens if I accidentally give too much insulin?

A. Believe it or not, this is not an uncommon mistake. If you've given too much insulin, contact your health care team. You'll need to monitor blood glucose levels every two to three hours. Set your alarm to wake you up through the night if necessary. You will need to provide extra food to prevent the blood glucose level from falling too low.

Q. My 14-year-old son has had diabetes for three years. He is now receiving three injections a day of NPH and Humalog. His last A1c was 7.9%. He is conscientious and responsible for his own diabetes care but still has low blood glucose episodes at night, two or three times per month. Would a pump help?

A. Giving insulin by continuous infusion with the pump may indeed reduce the risk of low blood glucose levels in the night, since the pump administers only very tiny amounts of insulin at a time. You describe your son as responsible and conscientious, both important attributes for pump therapy. To be successful, your son will be asked to become an expert carbohydrate counter and, hopefully, with your help, he'll be required to check his blood glucoses more frequently (that is, before and after meals and in the middle of the night) during the first few weeks of being on the pump. The use of a long-acting "peakless insulin" such as Lantus or Levemir together with a fast-acting insulin prior to meals may also reduce the risk of low blood glucose levels through the night.

> **Did You Know?**
> **Alcohol Swabbing**
>
> Most diabetes centers no longer include alcohol swabbing as part of their injection technique. There's no evidence to show that brief alcohol swabbing has any effect when people bathe regularly. Injection-site infections are exceptionally rare.

Q. My son is 12 years of age and has been on the pump for nearly 18 months. When he first went on the pump, his blood glucose concentrations were quite stable and his A1c dropped from 8.4% to 6.7%. However, during the last six months, his A1c has climbed to 8.1% and his blood glucose concentrations are all over the place. What is going on and what can I do?

A. The fact that his A1c dropped to 6.7% suggests that pump therapy can work well for your son. However, remember that pump therapy is just another way of giving insulin; it does not measure the blood glucose, and it only gives the amount of insulin that you have programmed it to provide. The primary principles of balancing food, insulin and exercise remain the same, and monitoring blood glucose before meals and snacks is the guide to this balance.

There are many reasons why your son's blood glucose control may have changed.

- If his diet has changed, you must ensure that the pump settings have been changed accordingly.
- If your child has grown or gained weight, his pump settings may need to be adjusted.
- If his activity has changed, especially if he has become more active with competitive athletics, his previous pump settings may be giving him too much insulin at some times and not enough at other times. You probably should do more blood glucose testing before, during and after the activity to provide you with the information needed to make appropriate changes to the pump settings.
- For insulin to do its job, it must be in good shape and get into the body appropriately. Make sure that the insulin in the reservoir is clear, that your son is changing his cannula and the attached catheter frequently enough, and that he is inserting the cannula into smooth and healthy sites.
- The most common reason for deterioration in blood glucose control on a pump is missed boluses. Check the bolus history on the pump and work out a system with your son to remind him to give his insulin at the right times.

In general, just because your son appears comfortable with the pump and its operation does not mean that you should totally back off. Stay in the loop so that you can help him to problem-solve.

The most common reason for deterioration in blood glucose control on a pump is missed boluses.

Chapter 5

Handling the Highs and Lows

It has been said that managing diabetes is a little like performing a complicated juggling act. Sometimes the ball drops. No matter how hard you try, it's impossible to keep the blood glucose in the target range all of the time. Sometimes it will be high, other times low. Often there is no explanation for the results.

This chapter will focus on hypoglycemia (low blood glucose; hyperglycemia (high blood glucose); prevention of diabetic ketoacidosis; and sick days, leading to loss of control of the diabetes.

> No matter how hard you try, it's impossible to keep the blood glucose in the target range all of the time. Sometimes it will be high, other times low. Often there is no explanation for the results.

Key Messages

- Although blood glucose levels may be outside of the desired target range at times, there are ways to limit the frequency and impact of this.

- During an illness (for example, the flu), people with type 1 diabetes need to take steps to prevent losing control of blood glucose levels (hypoglycemia and diabetic ketoacidosis).

- Caregivers need to feel confident about what to do in certain urgent situations that can come up in managing a child's diabetes.

Hypoglycemia (Low Blood Glucose)

Most people with type 1 diabetes experience low blood glucose episodes from time to time. Indeed, mild hypoglycemia that can be easily identified and treated, without too much interruption in activities, should be expected.

Low circulating blood glucose levels are due to an imbalance between the amount of glucose that enters the blood (either directly from food intake or from the stored glucose, or glycogen, in the liver) and the amount of glucose removed from the blood (for example, used by the brain and muscle cells).

In individuals without diabetes, the body turns off the supply of insulin whenever blood glucose levels are in the normal range. Therefore, low blood glucose never occurs in those with normal insulin secretion. However, episodes of low blood glucose can occur in people with diabetes because injected insulin cannot be "shut off" whenever blood glucose is at a normal or below normal level. Compared to insulin that is made in the body, injected insulin continues to work. As fast as the glucose enters the bloodstream, it then pushes it into the cells, causing the level of glucose in the blood to remain low until the person consumes carbohydrate.

It is because of this abnormal regulation of insulin and blood glucose in those with type 1 diabetes that close attention is needed to prevent, detect and treat hypoglycemia. Most **hypoglycemic events** are related to "predictable" events in self-care. Although all hypoglycemic episodes result from an imbalance between insulin action and glucose availability, there are three identifiable conditions under which hypoglycemia can be expected:

- **Too much insulin:** Sometimes children get the wrong type of insulin or take the wrong amount at the wrong time. Other times parents or teens do not make changes in the insulin dose when there are low glucose readings.

- **Not enough food:** This can happen easily enough — for example, when children get caught up in their activities and forget to eat, when toddlers sleep through snack time or when teens sleep through breakfast or skip a meal.

- **Too much unplanned activity:** This is the most frequent cause of hypoglycemia, because children aren't used to planning ahead before they jump into an active game like tag or soccer. That's why the blood glucose target range may need to be wider in younger children than in adults; it allows for more variability in activity.

Signs and Symptoms of Hypoglycemia

The earliest symptoms of low blood glucose are called early warning signs and may resemble the feelings many people experience when they've gone without food for a long time: they may feel hungry, tired and irritable, and they may even have a headache. These early warning signs tell us that the body needs glucose quickly. As the blood glucose continues to drop, other signs and symptoms may develop: shakiness, pale skin, cold sweat, dilated pupils and pounding heart. These result from the body's attempt to boost the blood glucose. Certain hormones — including glucagon, adrenaline, cortisol and others — urge our liver and muscles to convert stored glucose into glucose that can enter the bloodstream.

If not treated immediately, the early warning signs can worsen significantly, developing eventually into severe hypoglycemia, with confusion, coma and convulsions (called **neuroglycopenia**, or low glucose in the brain).

Although low blood glucose symptoms vary, each child tends to develop their own set of symptoms. After a few episodes, most parents and children learn to recognize hypoglycemia more quickly. It is important for parents and older children to explain the child's specific symptoms to

Signs and Symptoms: Hypoglycemia

Mild Hypoglycemia: Autonomic Symptoms
(Activated by the nervous system)
- Shakiness — "butterflies," feeling nervous for no reason
- Pounding heart
- Cold, clammy sweatiness
- Dilated pupils, "funny-looking" eyes
- Hunger, and sometimes nausea due to the hunger
- Change in skin color, paleness in the face

Moderate Hypoglycemia: Neuroglycopenic Symptoms
(Due to lack of glucose to the brain)
- Lack of energy — tired, weak, floppy
- Lack of concentration
- Mood change — for example, irritable, grouchy, impatient
- Blurred vision
- Poor sleep patterns — restlessness, crying out, sleepwalking or nightmares

teachers, coaches and other caregivers. Even young children can be taught to alert an adult to these symptoms by using a specific phrase such as "I feel funny" or "I need sugar." Hypoglycemia may be most difficult to detect in infants or toddlers, who are unable to describe their feelings.

When Does Hypoglycemia Happen?

Most people with type 1 diabetes experience low blood glucose episodes from time to time. Usually hypoglycemic episodes happen suddenly, over a period of minutes rather than hours. While they may occur at any time of the day or night, they happen most often when insulin is working at its peak.

HOW TO: Respond to Hypoglycemia

It's important to treat signs of hypoglycemia right away by following these steps.

1. **Check** the blood glucose level if hypoglycemia is suspected. If accompanied by symptoms of low blood glucose, even a blood glucose level lower than 110 mg/dL (6 mmol/L) should be treated.

2. **Treat** with a source of fast-acting sugar. These are made of just one or two sugar molecules. They are the quickest source of energy, as they are very rapidly digested. Typically, 10 to 15 grams of carbohydrate is the correct amount for children and teens. If in doubt, treat (for example, when you can't check the blood glucose level to confirm hypoglycemia).
   Note: Always have a source of fast-acting sugar available, such as juice or dextrose tablets. If you are going outside of the home with your child, make sure you always have this with you in an accessible place. When your child is somewhere without you, make sure another caregiver or the child themselves has convenient fast-acting sugar sources available.

3. **Wait** for the sugar to take effect. This is the hardest part. People who experience hypoglycemia can feel extremely hungry and scared. They are often tempted to continue to eat and drink until the symptoms go away. This may result in a high blood glucose level later in the day.

4. **Recheck** the blood glucose in 10 to 15 minutes. If it is still low, re-treat with a fast-acting carbohydrate.

5. **Try** to determine the cause of the low blood glucose event. If there is no apparent reason and a low has occurred at the same time the previous day, consider reducing the appropriate insulin by 10% the next day (see chapter 4 for insulin dose adjustment guidelines).

6. **Note** the blood glucose levels, time, response and possible cause of the hypoglycemic episode in your logbook.

Indeed, mild hypoglycemic episodes that are easily recognized and treated, without too much interruption in activities, should be expected. They can be seen as the price paid for good blood glucose control. Note that some people experience symptoms of hypoglycemia even when their blood glucose level is higher than 72 mg/dL (4 mmol/L). And if someone's blood glucose levels often run too high, they can even experience hypoglycemia signs and symptoms when their blood glucose level is in normal range.

Pro Tip

If a mild low blood glucose episode occurs just before a meal or snack, start the meal or snack immediately, beginning with some fast-acting sugar.

Hypoglycemia Treatment: Examples Based on Child's Weight

Weight	Less than 30 lbs (15 kg)	30–75 lbs (15–30 kg)	More than 60 lbs (30 kg)
Amount of carbohydrate required	5 g	10 g	15 g
Fast-acting sugars and their carbohydrate content (g)	1–1½ tsp (5–7 mL) sugar added to ¼ cup (60 mL) water (4–6 g)	2–3 Dex4 tabs (8–12 g)	4 Dex4 tabs or 1 Dex4 gel tube (16 g)
	1½ oz (45 mL) fruit juice (5 g)	3 oz (90 mL) fruit juice (10 g)	4 oz (125 mL) fruit juice (15 g)
	¼ cup (60 mL) chocolate milk (7 g)	⅓ cup (75 mL) chocolate milk (9 g)	½ cup (125 mL) chocolate milk (14 g)
	½ cup (125 mL) milk (6 g)	¾ cup (175 mL) milk (10 g)	1–1¼ cups (250–300 mL) milk (12–15 g)
	¼ cup (60 mL) regular soda (7 g)	⅓ cup (75 mL) regular soda (9 g)	½ cup (125 mL) regular soda (14 g)
	1–1½ tsp (5–7 mL) honey (5 g)	2 tsp (10 mL) honey (11 g)	1 tbsp (15 mL) honey (17 g)
	1–1½ tsp (5–7 mL) jam, jelly or maple syrup (4–6 g)	2–3 tsp (10–15 mL) jam, jelly or maple syrup (8–12 g)	1 tbsp (15 mL) jam, jelly or maple syrup (13 g)
	n/a	10–11 pieces Skittles candy (9–10 g)	15 pieces Skittles candy (14 g)

Reducing the Risk of Hypoglycemia

Low blood glucose episodes are not always preventable, but there are things you can do to keep them to a minimum and be prepared if they occur:

- Eat meals and snacks on time. A delay of half an hour or more can result in hypoglycemia.
- Make sure that the proper insulin dose is prepared and given. Even teens require close supervision with this task.
- Plan for extra activity with extra food or an insulin reduction. Set up a good communication system with teachers, coaches and other leaders. Set up realistic blood glucose targets for activity.
- Follow dose adjustment guidelines and decrease the insulin dose if the glucose level is low at the same time of day two days in a row, or three times in a week.
- Always have some form of quick-acting glucose close by and make sure everyone knows where it is. This includes having a source in the car for teens who are driving.
- Make sure teens are aware that drinking alcohol can cause delayed hypoglycemia.
- Always have a glucagon kit at home (see "About Glucagon," page 75). Review its use regularly. Take it with you on vacation. Replace it when it reaches its expiry date, and practice preparing it before you throw it out.
- Encourage your child to wear medical-alert identification and to carry a wallet card if older.

Pro Tip

If vigorous exercise is anticipated prior to the next meal or snack, or if the low blood glucose occurs during the night, the quick-acting carbohydrate should be followed with a longer-acting carbohydrate.

"False" Low Blood Glucose Episodes

Sometimes children feel anxious, nervous or tired and think it's due to low blood glucose when it isn't. There are many reasons for this. The nervousness a child feels over other things, such as exams, can be confused with hypoglycemia. And occasionally, the symptoms of high blood glucose are mistaken for hypoglycemia. A quick blood glucose check is the best way to find out whether the blood glucose is low. Once the blood glucose has been checked and it is clear that the result is not low, reassure your child that they can resume the activity. However, if in doubt, treat the symptoms.

Severe Hypoglycemia

Occasionally a severe hypoglycemic episode occurs when early symptoms of low blood glucose go undetected and untreated. Know what to look for and what to do in case a severe low blood glucose episode develops (see "Signs and Symptoms," below).

This is an emergency situation. Anyone showing signs of a severe hypoglycemic episode needs immediate help to increase their blood glucose. However, someone who is very drowsy, unconscious or having a convulsion or seizure must not be given juice or any other liquid by mouth, due to the risk of choking. Rather, the child should be turned onto their side to prevent choking, and glucagon (see "About Glucagon" below) should be injected. If a glucagon emergency kit is not available, an ambulance should be called and the child transported to the closest hospital emergency department, where either a glucose-containing solution will be injected intravenously or glucagon will be given. While you wait for the ambulance, honey or corn syrup may be rubbed on the lips, gums or lining of the child's mouth.

> Severe hypoglycemia is an emergency situation. Anyone showing signs of a severe hypoglycemic episode needs immediate help to increase their blood glucose.

Signs and Symptoms: Severe Hypoglycemia

- "Drunken-like behavior": slurred speech, staggering, confusion, combativeness
- Low energy — extremely tired, difficult to wake up
- Loss of consciousness
- Convulsions or seizures
- Temporary paralysis down one side of the body

About Glucagon

You will be taught how to inject glucagon should your child ever have low blood glucose and cannot swallow because of drowsiness or unconsciousness. Glucagon is a hormone that stimulates the liver to release its stored glucose into the bloodstream. It must be injected. When glucagon acts on the liver, the blood glucose level rises and the child begins to wake up within about 15 minutes.

Pro Tip

An injection of glucagon can only help. It can never be harmful. It is impossible to overdose on glucagon. Parents who think their child may need glucagon should play it safe and give the injection.

Families of all children with type 1 diabetes should have usable (not expired) glucagon on hand and know where it's kept and how to use it. A glucagon emergency kit consists of a small vial containing dry glucagon powder and a pre-filled glass syringe containing sterile diluting solution. The contents of the syringe and vial should be mixed only when they are about to be used. Keep the kit in an agreed-upon place so everyone can find it easily.

HOW TO: Prepare and Give Glucagon

1. Remove the flip-off seal from the bottle of glucagon.

2. Remove the needle protector from the syringe and inject the entire contents of the syringe into the vial of glucagon.

3. Shake the vial gently until the glucagon dissolves and the solution becomes clear. There is no need to remove the needle from the vial while shaking the bottle.

4. Using the same syringe, withdraw the solution from the vial. If the child is more than 5 years old, withdraw the full solution from the bottle (to the 1-mg mark on the syringe). If the child is 5 years or younger, withdraw half of the solution from the bottle (0.5-mg mark on the syringe).

5. Inject as you would insulin (same technique and spots).

Did You Know?
Preventing Another Episode

We know that one severe hypoglycemic episode makes the person with diabetes more susceptible to another episode in the next 24 to 48 hours. To prevent another episode, the appropriate insulin dose should be reduced by about 20% for at least the next day or two.

After the glucagon has been injected, check the blood glucose and observe the child carefully. Make sure the child is turned on their side to avoid choking. Usually, it takes about 5 to 20 minutes for the child to wake up. If this does not happen, the child should be taken to the closest hospital emergency department. Once the child is fully awake, offer some juice or a glucose-containing soda. Note: Diet sodas do not contain glucose and therefore will not reverse the symptoms of hypoglycemia. Recheck the blood glucose and notify the doctor.

Either the severe hypoglycemic episode or the use of glucagon can trigger nausea or vomiting, especially in children; they may be unable to eat or drink afterward. If this occurs:

- Recheck blood glucose levels immediately.
- If you are able to reach the doctor, they can advise you on whether to proceed to the hospital.
- If you cannot reach the doctor, go to the nearest hospital, even if the blood glucose levels are starting to rise.

CASE HISTORY
A Preventable Emergency

One day at about 10 a.m., we received a frantic call from the mother of a 16-year-old boy with type 1 diabetes who'd had the condition for more than 10 years. A single parent, she had come home from her night shift as a nurse to find her son unable to be woken in his bed. His blood glucose was "LO" on his meter when she checked. This had never happened before and she was in a state of severe panic. She was asked if she had glucagon at home and, if so, did she know how to use it. She answered yes to both questions. Our team member waited on the line while she gave the glucagon. When she returned to the phone, she was instructed to call 911 for the emergency medical services. They arrived within three minutes, checked his glucose, which was still very low, and gave him an intravenous injection of glucose. He woke up in minutes. They brought him to the hospital.

After more careful questioning, a few things emerged: first, he had been having quite a few early-morning low readings in the past few weeks and had not brought these to his mom's attention, nor made appropriate decreases in insulin dosage; second, he had been playing basketball the previous evening and had missed his bedtime snack because he was too tired; and third, his mom had given him the fluid in the glucagon syringe without mixing in the glucagon crystals before injection — so he had not gotten any glucagon.

Looking back on the episode, it's easy to determine what went wrong and how the episode might have been prevented:

1. *There had been indicators that his blood glucose was running low for some time before the episode, but he had not adjusted his insulin.*
2. *He had done vigorous exercise the night before.*
3. *He had skipped his late-evening snack on a day when it was more essential than most.*
4. *There was no one to prompt him to wake up on time and check his glucose.*
5. *When it came time to give the glucagon, Mom was so anxious that she failed to give the glucagon as she had been taught.*

Like most severe hypoglycemic events, this one was entirely preventable!

Mini-Dose Glucagon

Sometimes when children are sick they are unable or unwilling to drink and their blood glucose begins to drop. The guidelines that follow provide you with a way to respond to low blood glucose levels when your child is sick and unable to take glucose by mouth. By being prepared to inject tiny doses of glucagon at home when this situation occurs, you may be able to avoid an emergency room visit. Mini-dose glucagon increases the blood glucose level quite quickly and its action is brief. The dose may have to be repeated.

When to Use Mini-Dose Glucagon

You can safely inject your child with a small amount of glucagon if they are sick, if the blood glucose levels are persistently under 110 mg/dL (6 mmol/L), and they are vomiting or cannot take enough glucose by mouth to keep the blood glucose levels above 110 mg/dL (6 mmol/L).

Preparing and Giving Mini-Dose Glucagon

1. Inject the 1 mL of sterile diluting solution that is in the pre-filled glucagon syringe into the vial of glucagon and swirl the vial to mix the solution.

2. Determine how much mini-dose glucagon to give in the initial dose (see chart, page 79). *The maximum initial dose is 15 units.*

3. Use an insulin syringe (one capable of measuring small amounts) to measure the mini-dose glucagon solution from the vial. Ensure that the black plunger is in line with the markings on the side of the syringe.

4. Give the mini-dose glucagon injection in the same injection sites as you would with insulin.

After Giving the First Mini-Dose Glucagon Dose

1. Check your child's blood glucose after 15 minutes and then every 30 minutes until blood glucose is above 72 to 110 mg/dL (4 to 6 mmol/L).

2. If after 30 minutes the blood glucose level is still lower than 110 mg/dL (6 mmol/L), give your child another injection of mini-dose glucagon, but double the dose. *The maximum doubled dose is 30 units.*

3. Mini-dose glucagon can be given every 30 to 60 minutes.

4. Check the blood glucose at least every 30 minutes until it is over 110 mg/dL (6 mmol/L), then every hour until your child is able to take enough sugar by mouth to keep the blood glucose level in a safe range.

5. Keep the unused glucagon in the refrigerator for up to 24 hours.

6. Don't forget to get a replacement glucagon kit from your pharmacy.

How Much Mini-Dose Glucagon to Give

Age	Initial Dose*	Doubled Dose*	Example
Less than 2 years	2 units	4 units	If the child is 18 months old, give 2 units for the initial dose and 8 units for doses 2 to 5.
2–15 years	1 unit per year of age	2 units per year of age	If the child is 10 years old, give 10 units for the initial dose and 20 units for doses 2 to 5.
Over 15 years	15 units*	30 units*	If the child is 17 years old, give 15 units for the initial dose and 30 units for doses 2 to 5.

* The maximum initial dose of mini-dose glucagon is 15 units. The maximum doubled dose is 30 units.

Hyperglycemia (High Blood Glucose)

Parents of children with diabetes quickly discover that, no matter how much they know about this condition and no matter how hard they try to get excellent blood glucose results, the levels will be high from time to time. This is to be expected. Sometimes the reasons are obvious — a test done too soon after the last meal or snack, a lazy rainy day, an extra treat at a birthday party or some insulin leakage from an injection site. Sometimes the reason is less obvious; perhaps a bottle of insulin was inadvertently frozen, heated or ruined in some other way, and a fresh bottle is required.

Often, however, there's no obvious reason for the high level, which will seem unfair to those who invest a lot of time and effort in controlling blood glucose. But it's no one's fault. Rather, it's the result of an imperfect means of replacing insulin. Injecting insulin even three, four or more times a day does not restore the automatic blood glucose regulation that people without diabetes take for granted. There will be occasional highs regardless of how careful you are.

> There will be occasional highs regardless of how careful you are.

An isolated high blood glucose level — even one of 300 to 400 mg/dL (16 to 22 mmol/L) — is no cause for concern as long as the child feels well and there are no ketones in the urine. If high blood glucose levels persist, even in the absence of symptoms or ketones, an insulin adjustment may be required.

However, a high blood glucose level combined with ketones in the blood or urine, or with the signs and symptoms of high blood glucose, such as increased urination and thirst, indicates a need for immediate action. Additional short-acting or fast-acting insulin (NovoRapid, Humalog or Apidra) should be injected. In this situation, you should urgently contact your diabetes team; they will help you decide how much insulin to give. Failure to take action when the blood glucose level is high and ketones are present can lead to diabetic ketoacidosis, a preventable and life-threatening condition.

Diabetic Ketoacidosis

DKA is a serious situation that develops when there is a lack of insulin in the body. This may occur at the time of diagnosis (15% to 30% of children with newly diagnosed diabetes arrived in the emergency room with DKA) or if one of three situations arises:

1. Failure to get any or enough insulin

2. Failure to take sufficient extra insulin to cover the high glucose and ketone production caused by infection or another illness

3. Undetected or inappropriately managed pump failure (for those on insulin pumps)

With insufficient insulin available, blood glucose levels rise and excess glucose spills into the urine. The body then starts breaking down fat as an alternative supply of energy, and the child gets tired and starts to urinate and drink a lot. The ketones produced by fat breakdown are acidic, causing ketoacidosis. As more and more water is lost in the urine and as vomiting occurs with DKA, severe dehydration results. DKA can be avoided as long as the child gets all of the insulin all of the time and as long as illnesses are managed appropriately.

DKA usually develops over hours or days. For those using insulin pumps, DKA can happen more quickly than for those on a combination of fast and intermediate and/or long-acting insulin injections. This is because children on pumps use fast-acting insulin only and there is no background insulin in their system.

> DKA can be avoided as long as the child gets all of the insulin all of the time and as long as illnesses are managed appropriately.

Signs and Symptoms:
Diabetic Ketoacidosis

- High blood glucose levels and ketones in the urine or blood
- Excessive thirst
- Urinating much more often than usual and in larger amounts
- Sudden weight loss
- Complaints of stomach pains or nausea
- Vomiting
- Leg cramps
- A flushed appearance
- Headache
- Dehydration: dry mouth and tongue, sore throat, dark circles under the eyes
- Deep, heavy breathing; fruity-smelling breath
- Drowsiness leading in time to unconsciousness

Preventing DKA

Since one of the main reasons for developing DKA is failure to get enough insulin, parents must ensure that children and teens are getting the right amount of insulin at the right time. This responsibility is too much for a young child to assume alone. The other high-risk time for developing DKA is when the body is under stress due to fever — during an infection or flu, for example. These common conditions can become life-threatening if they are not adequately managed by the family with the support of their health care team. Become very familiar with the sick-day guidelines that follow. If you are taking a vacation, don't leave home without them.

Sick Days

Children with diabetes do not experience more illnesses than their nondiabetic friends, and they should not miss more school days because of their diabetes. An otherwise healthy person with well-controlled diabetes has normal resistance to infection. When diabetes is adequately controlled, injuries are not slow to heal. However, while illness may not be more likely or more difficult to treat in a person with diabetes, illness may upset the blood glucose balance.

When children with diabetes get sick, their blood glucose often goes high and ketones may show in the urine or blood. Illness is a stress to the body, and stress creates a demand for more insulin. People without diabetes automatically make more insulin at such times. Children with diabetes do not. Therefore, on a sick day, the usual amount of insulin may not be enough, and monitoring may show high blood glucose, with or without ketones. At such times, you may need to increase the insulin dose, even though the appetite may be poor, to prevent hyperglycemia and DKA.

Although all illnesses in people with diabetes must be taken seriously, not all illnesses make the blood glucose go up. In fact, illnesses like diarrhea may be accompanied by low blood glucose levels. Careful monitoring of blood glucose levels and urinary or blood ketones will help determine the effect of each illness and the appropriate response.

Pro Tip

We highly recommend the influenza vaccination each year for all people with type 1 diabetes.

What to Do When a Child with Diabetes Is Ill

- Check the blood glucose and urinary or blood ketone levels every two to four hours around the clock.

- Continue administering insulin. *Never miss a dose*, even if your child may not be eating well. Due to the physical stress of the illness, blood glucose levels likely will increase and cause ketones to form. Thus, more insulin may be needed, rather than less. If the glucose levels decrease, less (but never no) insulin may be required. Remember that insulin is always required to prevent the breakdown of body fat into ketones.

- Closely supervise blood glucose monitoring and insulin injections. Do not leave your child on their own to manage their diabetes when they are ill. Consider taking over routines for teens with diabetes who are doing their own monitoring and insulin administration.
- Be sure to treat the underlying illness that is upsetting diabetes control. Give the medications prescribed. Acetaminophen in the usual doses for fever or pain is safe unless your doctor says otherwise.
- Avoid dehydration. Drink extra sugar-free fluids and follow sick-day management to ensure carbohydrate intake.

Insulin Management during Illness

When children and teens get sick, they still need insulin at their usual times. In fact, they may require extra injections of fast-acting insulin as often as every four hours, if they show high blood glucose and urine or blood ketones. To decide how much insulin to give, check the blood glucose and urine or blood ketones every four hours and consult the chart below each time. As well, follow the chart for guidance on how much to reduce normal insulin dosages with low blood glucose levels during illness.

Small children and children who have been diagnosed in the last six months to a year tend to be sensitive to insulin: in this situation, you may want to choose a dose at the lower end of the range to begin and then go by your experience.

Contact your diabetes team immediately if you need help following these guidelines.

Blood Glucose	Urine Ketones	Blood Ketones	What to Do with the Insulin Dosage
<110 mg/dL (6 mmol/L)	Negative or positive	0.0–3.0	Reduce normal insulin dose by at least 10%–20%. Encourage sugar-containing fluids. May be time to use mini-dose glucagon.
110–230 mg/dL (6–13 mmol/L)	Negative or positive	0.0–3.0	Give the usual insulin at normal time. **Do not** give extra insulin. Recheck in 4 hours.
>230 mg/dL (13 mmol/L)	Negative or small positive (+)	0.0–0.6	Give more fast-acting insulin (e.g., Humalog or NovoRapid — up to 10% of the total daily dose) **now**. Recheck in 4 hours.
>230 mg/dL (13 mmol/L)	Moderate or large positive (++, +++)	0.7–3.0	Give more fast-acting insulin (e.g., Humalog or NovoRapid — at least 10%–20% of the total daily dose) **now**. Recheck in 4 hours.

Calculating Total Daily Dose (TDD)

Add up all doses of slow-acting and fast-acting insulin that your child is currently taking on a regular day (if using a sliding scale, this does not include your correction doses):

Total intermediate- or long-acting (for example, NPH, Lantus, Levemir) + total fast-acting (for example, Humalog, NovoRapid) = _____ (TDD)

10% of TDD: _____

20% of TDD: _____

Planning Meals on Sick Days

Often a child's appetite decreases with illness. If your child is not able to eat solid food, make sure they have drinks that contain carbohydrate. This will help to:

- Get enough liquids
- Have enough energy to fight the infection
- Keep blood glucose levels in a healthy and safe range

If Your Child Is Counting Carbohydrates

- Try to keep following the meal plan. Your child still needs carbohydrates to prevent a low blood glucose episode.
  - If your child has a hard time eating solid food, you can give them drinks that contain carbohydrate. Aim for 10 to 15 grams of carbohydrate every hour. This will replace the amount of carbohydrate your child would normally have during that day (see examples below).
  - If needed, spread carbohydrates evenly throughout the day.

For example, if your child has 42 grams of carbohydrate for breakfast and 15 grams for morning snack, the total for the morning is 57 grams of carbohydrate. This amount of carbohydrate can be spread out between breakfast time and lunch if your child cannot eat the total carbohydrate amount at the normal times.

Pro Tip

For children and teens on pumps, the total daily insulin dose can be found in the memory of the pump. This amount includes both the amount of basal and bolus insulin that the pump delivers.

Examples of Liquids That Contain 10 to 15 grams of Carbohydrate

- ½ cup (125 mL) of juice
- Approximately ⅓ of a 12-oz (355 mL) can of regular ginger ale
- ½ popsicle
- ¼ cup (60 mL) of regular Jell-O
- ½ cup (125 mL) of Gatorade

Illness Management with the Insulin Pump

- **Important:** Vomiting along with high blood glucose and ketones must always be treated as a pump failure until proven otherwise. Discontinue the pump immediately, ensure mechanical problems have been ruled out and perform a full infusion set change. In the meantime, use a pen or syringe to inject fast-acting insulin equal to the amount of 10% to 20% of the total daily dose (basal plus bolus).

- During illness, the usual correction dose suggested by the pump may not be enough, and one or more additional boluses equal to 10% to 20% of the total daily dose may be necessary. If food is being eaten at this time, this correction dose will need to be added to the amount of insulin needed for the carbohydrate. (See chart and information on page 64 regarding when and how to calculate extra bolus doses). **Important:** In this situation, you should *not* use the Bolus Wizard/EZ BG feature on the pump.

- With an illness where there are consistently high blood glucose levels, the basal rate may also need to be temporarily increased. Start with an increase of 20%; depending on the results, further increases may need to be made.

- If vomiting occurs more than twice within a four-hour period, call the diabetes team for advice. You may need to go to the closest emergency department.

- Check the blood glucose and ketone levels at least every four hours and consult the chart below to take recommended action.

Blood Glucose	Blood Ketone Level	Urine Ketone Level	Action to Take with the Insulin Pump
≤72 mg/dL (4.0 mmol/L)	Any amount	Negative or positive	Decrease pre-meal bolus dose and/or program a lower temporary basal rate by 20%–50%. Encourage your child to drink sugar-containing fluids in order to maintain blood glucose in the 110–180 mg/dL (6–10 mmol/L) range. If your child is vomiting, contact your diabetes team.
72–230 mg/dL (4.0–13 mmol/L)	<0.6	Negative or positive (any amount)	Take usual insulin dose (same as for non-sick day).
>230 mg/dL (13 mmol/L)	0.6–1.5	Negative or small positive (+)	Take 10% of TDD now, *in addition to* the dose needed for carbohydrate.
>230 mg/dL (13 mmol/L)	1.5–3.0	Moderate (++) to large (+++) positive	Take 20% of TDD now, *in addition to* the dose needed for carbohydrate.

Surgery

Most operations do not present problems for someone with diabetes, as long as careful attention is paid to blood glucose control before, during and after surgery. Surgery under local anesthesia usually does not require hospital admission. However, it is important that meals not be missed. Dentists, for example, should be told about the diabetes, and appointments for tooth extraction or root canal work should be scheduled so they don't interfere with meal or snack times.

If surgery under general anesthetic is required, hospital admission may be necessary and a physician experienced in the management of type 1 diabetes should be involved. Admission may be either the day before surgery or on the day of the procedure.

Q & A

Did You Know?

Smearing Honey

People sometimes smear honey in the mouth of a person with diabetes who is unable to swallow. The big risk of giving an unconscious person anything by mouth is that they may choke on it. Smearing honey on the lips or between the gums and cheek of an unconscious person with diabetes is better than trying to pour juice or force a hard candy into the mouth. But using glucagon is the best way to reverse a severe hypoglycemic episode rapidly.

Q. How many hypoglycemic episodes are too many?

A. The occasional mild to moderate low blood glucose episode — one that can be easily treated with juice — is to be expected, perhaps once or twice a week. However, these mild episodes can interrupt the school day or other activities and make it difficult for the child to concentrate for the following half hour or so. Prevent them as best you can, and respond to them quickly. Frequent lows need to be addressed with a change to the regimen. For example, if the teacher notices that your child is cranky everyday at 11:30 a.m. and low blood glucose is confirmed, it's time to reexamine the meal plan or insulin dose and make a change.

Q. What are the long-term effects of a severe low?

A. The greatest long-term effect is the fear that the child will have another severe hypoglycemic episode. This is a very real fear for many parents, siblings and children with diabetes, and it can cause a reluctance to keep trying to maintain good blood glucose control. This psychological setback is the only real long-term impact, because the body works very hard to protect the brain during events like this. Mildly delayed intellectual development has been noted in infants who experienced repeated episodes of severe hypoglycemia in the first three to five years of life.

Q. Is it possible to get diabetic ketoacidosis from eating too much glucose?

A. No. The worst that can happen is high blood glucose (hyperglycemia), which is undesirable but not the life–threatening condition of DKA. The only cause of DKA is a lack of insulin.

Q. Is it all right to give my child cough syrup and other medicines?

A. The U.S. Food and Drug Administration and Health Canada suggest that no oral cough or cold medications be given to very young children (FDA under 2 years of age; Health Canada under 6 years of age). If your child is older than 2 or 6 years and there is a cough syrup you find effective for your child, by all means use it as directed. The glucose content of the prescribed dose is probably minimal. However, if you're worried about the glucose in medications, ask your pharmacist to suggest preparations that are glucose-free.

Children with diabetes don't require medicine more often than other children. However, if the doctor prescribes a course of antibiotics, for example, it's important to finish the prescription, even if blood glucose levels begin to rise. Many parents mistakenly think the antibiotics are the cause of the blood glucose increase, but, in fact, the illness is probably causing stress on the body, leading to higher glucose levels.

There are medications containing steroids — such as prednisone, sometimes prescribed for children with asthma — that actually do cause blood glucose to rise. These drugs can create a need for much more insulin, but they should not be withheld if they're needed. Be prepared to increase the insulin dose.

If you're worried about the glucose in medications, ask your pharmacist to suggest preparations that are glucose-free.

Q. Older children can treat mild hypoglycemia with dextrose tablets or hard candies. What would you suggest for infants and toddlers?

A. Clearly, hard candies and dextrose tablets are inappropriate for young children. Depending on the child's weight, $1\frac{1}{2}$ to 3 oz (45 to 90 mL) of juice or $\frac{1}{2}$ to $\frac{3}{4}$ cup (125 to 175 mL) of milk in a bottle or cup would work. Some parents keep a tube of cake frosting handy for treating mild hypoglycemia.

Q. I read that the symptoms of hypoglycemia or diabetic ketoacidosis can be confused with drunkenness. Is that true?

A. It's true. The slurred speech, confusion, staggering and fatigue of hypoglycemia can look like drunken behavior. DKA may also be mistaken for drunkenness because the breath can smell a bit fruity, which can be confused with the smell of alcohol. However, what happens more often is that a person with diabetes has a couple of drinks and then begins to go low. (Alcohol causes low blood glucose if food isn't eaten at the same time.) A bystander who is unaware of the diabetes may smell alcohol on the breath and decide that the person is drunk. This is another good reason for someone with diabetes to wear a medical-alert bracelet.

A bystander who is unaware of the diabetes may smell alcohol on the breath and decide that the person is drunk. This is another good reason for someone with diabetes to wear a medical-alert bracelet.

Chapter 6

A Word about Type 2 Diabetes

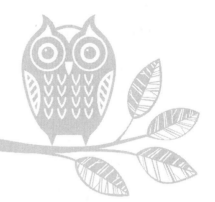

Type 2 diabetes in the most common type of diabetes in adults. Over the past 30 years, there has been a gradual increase in the number of children with type 2 diabetes. The rates of type 2 diabetes vary by the ethnicity of the child and are very much influenced by the presence of childhood overweight or obesity. The vast majority of youngsters developing type 2 diabetes are adolescent at the time of diagnosis. In this chapter, we briefly highlight the differences between types 1 and 2 diabetes and provide a framework for managing type 2 diabetes.

Key Messages

- Type 2 diabetes is increasing in frequency in children and teens, but remains much less common than type 1.

- Children with certain risk factors — such as being overweight or obese; a strong family history of type 2 diabetes; or belonging to a certain ethnic group — are at an increased likelihood of developing type 2 diabetes.

- The increasing incidence of type 2 diabetes in children worldwide parallels very closely the rise in childhood obesity.

- Lifestyle changes, including increasing exercise and optimizing healthy food choices, are an essential part of the management of type 2 diabetes and should be undertaken not only by the child, but by the entire family.

- Screening for complications associated with type 2 diabetes should start at the time of diagnosis in order to detect early reversible changes.

In the United States, the incidence of type 2 diabetes is between about 8 and 12 per 100,000 children and teens. In Canada, the incidence of type 2 diabetes is about 1.5 per 100,000 children and teens per year, except in Manitoba,

> The management of type 2 diabetes involves significant lifestyle changes and following through with new day-to-day routines.

which has an incidence over 12.5. These figures compare to about 25 cases per 100,000 children per year developing type 1 diabetes in both the U.S. and Canada.

The management of type 2 diabetes involves significant lifestyle changes and following through with new day-to-day routines. Commitment on the part of the whole family is essential and can successfully support children and teens to make changes that are beneficial for everyone in the home.

What Causes Type 2 Diabetes?

Type 2 diabetes is not an autoimmune condition like type 1 diabetes. In type 1 diabetes, the body produces an immune response that attacks and destroys the insulin-producing cells in the pancreas (beta cells). Antibodies to specific islet-cell (beta-cell) proteins are evidence of the autoimmune response. In type 2 diabetes, on the other hand, these immune responses are not present. Instead, the body responds less well to insulin (this is called insulin resistance). Insulin resistance means that

Comparison of Type 1 and Type 2 Diabetes

There are important differences in how the different types of diabetes present that may alert your doctor to a diagnosis of type 2 diabetes.

	Type 1 Diabetes	Type 2 Diabetes
Age of presentation	Can occur at any age after 6 months of age	Most commonly occurs in children older than 10 years of age and those who have gone through puberty
Family history	While there is an increased risk in families with a first-degree relative with type 1 diabetes, commonly there will not be a family history of diabetes	Usually there is a family history of type 2 diabetes or gestational diabetes (diabetes in the mother during pregnancy)
Ethnicity	Seen in all ethnicities	Increased risk in populations such as Aboriginal Americans and Canadians, Hispanics, African-Americans, African-Canadians and Asians
Body weight	Not associated with a particular body weight	Often associated with the child being overweight or obese
Diabetes ketoacidosis at presentation	20%–30% of children will present with diabetic ketoacidosis at initial diagnosis	~10% of children will present with diabetic ketoacidosis at initial diagnosis

more and more insulin needs to be produced in the body to have the same glucose-lowering effect. Initially the body tries to compensate for this insulin resistance by producing more insulin. However, over time, the insulin-producing beta cells start to fail and cannot produce enough insulin to keep the blood glucose levels in the normal range.

Risk Factors for Type 2 Diabetes

- Having a family member with type 2 diabetes
- Having a weight above the recommended weight range (greater than or equal to the 95th percentile for the child's age and gender)
- Being more sedentary or less active
- Being from a certain ethnic group (such as Aboriginal American or Canadian, African-American, African-Canadian, Asian or Hispanic)
- Having a mother who had diabetes during pregnancy (gestational diabetes)
- Taking certain medications, such as antipsychotics or glucocorticoids (steroids)
- Having certain conditions, such as polycystic ovarian syndrome or nonalcoholic fatty liver disease (NAFLD)

It is recommended that children with more than one of these risk factors be regularly screened for the development of type 2 diabetes by testing a fasting (first thing in the morning before eating) blood glucose level every two years.

> **Did You Know?**
> **Asymptomatic Diabetes**
>
> A sizable proportion, perhaps even the majority, of teens presenting with type 2 diabetes do so asymptomatically (that is, the diabetes is detected by screening rather than checking blood glucose levels in response to signs or symptoms).

How Does Type 2 Diabetes Present in Children and Teens?

As the blood glucose levels increase and exceed the kidney's ability to reabsorb the excess glucose, children will often experience increased urine production (polyuria) and increased thirst (polydipsia). In type 2 diabetes, these symptoms can often be quite subtle and easily overlooked. As a result, these high blood glucose symptoms can occur for many weeks or months prior to the child being diagnosed with diabetes.

Similar to type 1 diabetes, there can be other associated symptoms, such as weight loss and increased tiredness. As well, because of the increased level of glucose in the urine, girls in particular may present with yeast or bladder infections.

> High blood glucose symptoms can occur for many weeks or months prior to the child being diagnosed with diabetes.

Along with these typical symptoms of diabetes, in type 2 diabetes, there sometimes can be unique signs of the body being resistant to insulin:

- A dark, velvety rash usually seen on the back of the neck, in the armpits or in the creases of the skin; this is called acanthosis nigricans and is a sign that the body is resistant to insulin
- In girls, irregular menstrual periods
- In girls, increase in body hair (hirsutism)

Diabetic Ketoacidosis and Severe Dehydration

Although it is uncommon, children and teens with type 2 diabetes can sometimes be diagnosed with diabetic ketoacidosis. This occurs when the insulin-producing cells (beta cells) fail and do not produce sufficient insulin to provide energy to the body, so that fat breakdown occurs instead. In other children with type 2 diabetes, extremely high blood glucose levels can lead to severe dehydration, increasing the concentration of the blood and sometimes resulting in a state of reduced consciousness. This condition is referred to as a hyperosmolar hyperglycemic state.

Although many children with type 2 diabetes present with gradual symptoms over time, given these serious but rare conditions, it is still important that any child suspected to potentially have type 2 diabetes be assessed by a physician in a timely manner.

Making the Diagnosis

In children with symptoms suggestive of type 2 diabetes, the diagnosis can be made by measuring a high blood glucose level at any time of the day. The diagnosis can also be made if there are no symptoms but two high blood glucose measurements have been taken. High blood glucose levels can be measured in three different ways:

- A fasting blood glucose level greater than or equal to 126 mg/dL (7 mmol/L)
- A random blood glucose level greater than or equal to 200 mg/dL (11.1 mmol/L)
- A blood glucose level greater than or equal to 200 mg/dL (11.1 mmol/L) after a two-hour oral glucose tolerance test; an oral glucose tolerance test is when the blood glucose level is measured two hours after the child is given a special sugary liquid to drink

Managing Type 2 Diabetes

Many of the basic skills required to manage type 2 diabetes are the same as for type 1 diabetes. It is important to monitor blood glucose levels and to record the readings in order to be able to assess the effectiveness of the treatment (see chapter 2). The target blood glucose range before meals for children with type 2 diabetes is between 72 and 126 mg/dL (4 and 7 mmol/L), with an A1c level (a measure of the average blood glucose level over the three previous months) of less than or equal to 7%. Unlike children with type 1 diabetes, not all children with type 2 diabetes need to be treated with insulin. However, it is important to recognize that insulin treatment for some may still be needed to achieve target blood glucose control either immediately at diagnosis or at a later point in time.

Lifestyle Management

For all children with type 2 diabetes, optimizing nutrition and exercise are key first steps in the management plan. Increased activity can decrease insulin resistance and reduce blood glucose levels. For children between 12 and 18 years of age, participation in at least 60 minutes of moderate to vigorous physical activity each day is recommended. At least three days a week this activity should be at a vigorous level.

- Moderate-intensity physical activity should cause you to sweat a little and breathe harder. Examples include bike riding and swimming.

- Vigorous-intensity physical activity should cause you to sweat and be out of breath. Examples include running and in-line skating.

Pro Tip

Choosing activities that teens will find fun, rather than a burden, is a key step in trying to maintain long-term lifestyle changes.

There are different ways to achieve these activity goals. Examples of how to fit extra exercise into everyday activities include: walking part or all of the way to school; walking the dog; or having the whole family participate in extra activities, such as going to the park, on the weekend.

In addition to increasing the level of activity, it is important to reduce the amount of time spent being sedentary or sitting indoors each day. One recommendation is to limit screen time — on computers, playing video games or watching television — to no more than two hours a day.

Making healthy food choices and maintaining a well-balanced diet can also lead to reduced demand for insulin from the pancreas and can decrease blood glucose readings.

A dietitian on your diabetes team can help identify specific nutrition goals and design a personalized meal plan. Similar to increasing activity levels, having a healthy diet is most successful when the entire family incorporates these principles into their daily practice.

Healthy lifestyle tips to consider include:

- Eat three regular meals each day, including breakfast. Skipping meals often can lead to making poor food choices later in the day, when your child is hungry. Eating regularly can help avoid big fluctuations in insulin release from the pancreas and result in more stable blood glucose levels.

- Sit down at the table as a family to eat. When the child eats in front of the television, in their room or by themselves, it often results in an increased amount of food being eaten.

- Have a variety of food at each meal, including vegetables and fruit, meat or alternative, and whole-grain breads and cereals.

- Avoid sugary drinks, including juice and sodas. These contain a lot of carbohydrate and calories with little nutritional value. Drinking water is best, and eating whole fruit is preferable to drinking juice.

- Limit the amount of fast-food products and high-fat foods eaten.

- Avoid eating too many salty foods or adding too much salt.

Making small changes to the everyday eating pattern and incorporating daily healthy food choices are essential to achieving and maintaining long-term lifestyle changes. As this can be difficult, it is important that the entire family helps to support and adopt these changes.

Medication

Many children with type 2 diabetes may find it difficult to achieve their blood glucose targets with lifestyle changes alone. In addition to insulin, which may be needed, other medications are prescribed to children with type 2 diabetes (see table, page 95).

Metformin (trade name Glucophage) is the most commonly used medication in children with type 2 diabetes. It is given as a pill, usually twice a day. It works by making the body more sensitive to the action of its own insulin and reduces the amount of glucose produced by the liver. In some, it can also diminish appetite. Through these effects, it decreases the blood glucose levels. Importantly, it does not cause low blood glucose levels (hypoglycemia) unless used with other medications, such as insulin, or if a teen is drinking alcohol. The most common side effect of metformin is abdominal discomfort, sometimes with associated nausea, loss of appetite or loose bowel movements. To reduce the likelihood of these side effects, your doctor may start with a low dose of metformin and slowly increase the dose over time. Taking the medication with food can also reduce the chance of these abdominal symptoms occurring.

There are several different other categories of medications used to treat type 2 diabetes. Insulin can play an important role in the management of type 2 diabetes. It may be used at the time of diagnosis if the blood glucose levels are very high. Alternatively, it may be added to other treatment options (such as metformin) if target blood glucose and A1c levels cannot be achieved. Depending on the child's blood glucose control, sometimes once daily long-acting basal insulin is used alone. For other children, however, multiple daily injections of insulin may be needed.

> Depending on the child's blood glucose control, sometimes once daily long-acting basal insulin is used alone. For other children, however, multiple daily injections of insulin may be needed.

Class of Medication	Examples: Generic Name (U.S.; Canadian [if different])	How It Is Given	How It Works
Sodium-glucose transporter 2 inhibitors	• Canagliflozin (Invokana) • Empagliflozin (Jardiance) • Dapagliflozin (Forxiga)	Oral medication	Increases glucose loss in urine, leading to lower blood glucose levels
DPP-4 inhibitors	• Sitagliptin (Januvia) • Saxagliptin (Onglyza) • Linagliptin (Tradjenta) • Alogliptin (Nesina)	Oral medication	Increases insulin release from pancreas, but only when blood glucose levels are increased
GLP-1 receptor antagonists	• Exenatide (Byetta) • Liraglutide (Victoza) • Albiglutide (Eperzan) • Dulaglutide (Trulicity)	Subcutaneous injection	Increases insulin release from pancreas, but only when blood glucose levels are increased
Alpha-glucosidase inhibitors	• Acarbose (Precose; Prandase)	Oral medication	Slows the breakdown of carbohydrate to sugar in the intestine
Sulfonylureas*	• Gliclazide (Diamicron) • Glimepiride (Amaryl) • Glyburide (Micronase, Diabeta, Euglucon)	Oral medication	Stimulates beta cells in the pancreas to produce more insulin
Thiazolidinediones	• Rosiglitazone (Avandia) • Pioglitazone (Actos)	Oral medication	Makes cells more sensitive to insulin to improve cells' ability to use glucose

* May be available under more than one brand name.

Other medication options are mostly used in adults with type 2 diabetes, with limited experience in children. In the future, however, some of these may more commonly be used in children with type 2 diabetes. The table on page 95 gives some examples of these medications. This table does not include all the different brands of medications, as this continually changes over time.

The Importance of Getting to Target

Children with type 2 diabetes are at increased risk for long-term complications over time.

As with type 1 diabetes, the goals of getting the blood glucose levels into target range are to improve short-term symptoms (such as increased thirst and urination) and reduce the risk of long-term complications. This is especially important with type 2 diabetes, as children with this type of diabetes are at increased risk for long-term complications over time, as well as at the time of diagnosis. Because these complications can sometimes occur very early, screening needs to start at the time of diagnosis.

Screening for long-term complications includes regular assessment of:

- Blood cholesterol levels
- Blood pressure
- Kidneys (nephropathy screening), to look for evidence of protein in the urine
- Eyes (retinopathy screening), to assess the blood vessels in the back of the eye (in the **retina**)
- Nerves (neuropathy screening), to evaluate for numbness, pain and normal tendon reflexes

Further details about screening for diabetes complications can be found in chapter 13.

Although type 2 diabetes often is diagnosed incidentally or has a milder course than type 1 diabetes, it has serious long-term ramifications with respect to early-onset and severe cardiovascular disease. The aim for monitoring for the complications and associated conditions is to detect the symptoms early, before there are long-term irreversible changes. With glucose control in target and careful, regular screening, the long-term outcome for teens and children with type 2 diabetes can be excellent.

Other Associated Conditions

In type 2 diabetes, it is important to screen for associated conditions that can develop. These include:

- **Nonalcoholic fatty liver disease:** NAFLD occurs when there is an accumulation of fatty deposits in the liver. If the condition progresses over time, it can lead to scarring (fibrosis) in the liver, which can affect liver function. This will be monitored by testing an enzyme from the liver once a year. Management of this condition includes making lifestyle changes, in particular choosing healthy food options.

- **Polycystic ovarian syndrome (PCOS):** In girls, type 2 diabetes can be associated with PCOS. Symptoms include irregular or absent menstrual periods, increased acne, and hair growth on the face, chest or back. Screening for these symptoms is done yearly in post-pubertal girls with type 2 diabetes. While lifestyle changes can help with these symptoms, medications are sometimes recommended if these symptoms persist.

Q & A

Q. My teen needs to start taking insulin to manage her diabetes. Does this mean she now has type 1, not type 2, diabetes?

A. No, this does not mean she has type 1 diabetes. She still has type 2 diabetes, but now her blood glucose levels are being managed with insulin, likely in combination with an oral medication and lifestyle modifications. Sometimes insulin is needed temporarily to manage blood glucose when children are first diagnosed with type 2 diabetes, and often it is needed after they have had type 2 diabetes for a longer period of time. Regardless, type 1 and type 2 diabetes are currently classified as two separate conditions, since they have very different causes.

> Helping your family members to be more active and make healthy choices around eating can have a positive effect on weight, which, in turn, could improve how sensitive their body is to insulin.

Q. My teen has type 2 diabetes. Is there anything I can do to try to prevent my other children from developing it as well?

A. Although your other children are at greater risk for developing type 2 diabetes, this doesn't mean that they will inevitably develop this condition. Helping your family members to be more active and make healthy choices around eating can have a positive effect on weight, which, in turn, could improve how sensitive their body is to insulin. This could then either put off, or hopefully even prevent, the diagnosis of type 2 diabetes.

Chapter 7

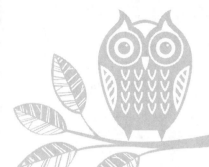

Making Meals Work

For some families, planning meals is the trickiest part of diabetes management. At first, you may look at food very differently than you did before. Many parents ask: Will my child's or teen's food intake need to be changed? The answer to that is that it depends.

In this chapter, we review the important things to consider when planning meals and snacks for children and teens with type 1 diabetes; however, the foundation is the same healthy, balanced diet that is recommended for all children.

Terminology

Many people associate the word *diet* with weight loss or restrictive eating plans, but, in fact, *diet* simply refers to the foods and drinks a person regularly consumes.

Key Messages

The main nutrition goals are:

- To promote normal growth and development by eating a healthy, balanced and age-appropriate diet.
- To accurately match insulin to food in order to help achieve blood glucose targets.
- To satisfy appetite and encourage a healthy, positive relationship with food.
- To support cultural dietary preferences.

The meal plan should be easy to follow, incorporate your child's or teen's likes and dislikes, and suit your family's lifestyle. As with other areas of diabetes management, the goal is to fit the diabetes into your child's life, not the other way around.

If any changes to your child's diet are needed, it is suggested that your whole family make them together, as it is much easier for your child if they are not singled out. To avoid frustration and conflict around food, the same rules should apply to everyone in your household. For some families, this will mean that few changes need to be made, while for others, more significant adjustments will likely be advised. Rest assured that you do not need to make these changes all at once or immediately at diagnosis. Together with your dietitian, you can set realistic goals to ensure this transition is successful.

Food Guides

The food guide MyPlate, developed by the U.S. Department of Agriculture, is a tool that describes how to achieve a healthy, balanced diet. The Canadian equivalent is Eating Well with Canada's Food Guide. Similar tools are available in other countries to help guide healthy eating. These food guides provide a road map to healthy eating, dividing foods into four or five food groups. For optimal health, we all need to eat a variety of foods from the food groups in certain quantities. A good rule of thumb is to include items from three to four food groups for meals and two food groups for snacks.

Following the principles of these food guides will help ensure that your child or teen is getting adequate energy, vitamins, minerals and other nutrients. You may already be familiar with your country's food guide; if not, your dietitian will help guide you through this resource.

You can find detailed information on the MyPlate guidelines at ChooseMyPlate.gov. You can download a copy of Eating Well with Canada's Food Guide at www.canada.ca/en/health-canada/services/canada-food-guides.html.

Macronutrients and Micronutrients

Let's begin with some basic nutrition concepts. The foods we eat provide many nutrients. The three main nutrients that provide us with energy, called **macronutrients**, are carbo-hydrate, protein and fat. You will see throughout this chapter that an emphasis is placed on learning about carbohydrate; however, these macronutrients are all important to your diet. Vitamins and minerals are **micronutrients**, which means they are only required in small amounts.

Macronutrients

These are the nutrients that are required in large amounts; they provide the energy needed to maintain body functions and carry out the activities of daily life:

- Carbohydrate
- Protein
- Fat

Did You Know?
Food Is Not Medicine

While nutrition is a very important part of diabetes management, it is important to remember that food is not medicine. While things may seem overwhelming at first, the presence of diabetes should not take the joy and pleasure out of eating.

Micronutrients

These are needed in very small amounts, but each is essential for a specific role in bodily function:

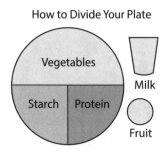

How to Divide Your Plate

- **Vitamins:** including vitamins A, B group, C, D, E and K
- **Minerals:** for example, iron, calcium, magnesium, zinc

Your child's or teen's nutritional requirements are no different than before they were diagnosed with diabetes. Their bodies need a combination of these macro- and micronutrients to grow and develop and to maintain optimal health. When planning meals, aim to make your plate look like the diagram at left.

How Foods Affect Blood Glucose Levels

Carbohydrate has the biggest and most direct impact on blood glucose, while protein and fat have a smaller effect. For this reason, special attention is given to the type, timing and amount of carbohydrate foods in your child's or teen's meal plan.

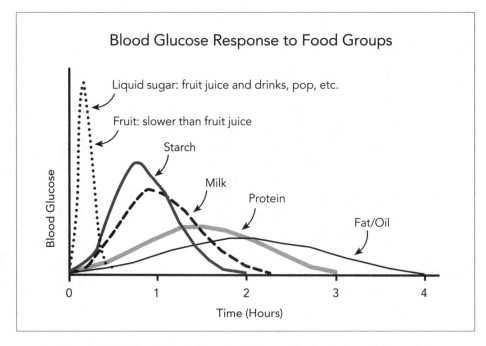

Source: BC Children's Hospital (www.bcchildrens.ca/endocrinology-diabetes-site/documents/glycemic.pdf)

Carbohydrate

Carbohydrate is an essential source of energy. It is important for our muscles, brain and nerves to work properly. Many carbohydrate foods are also rich in vitamins and minerals, making them an important part of the diet. Carbohydrate breaks down into glucose in the body and therefore is the macronutrient that will most directly raise blood glucose levels.

The table below offers examples of some foods that contain carbohydrate:

Grains and Starches	Fruits and Vegetables	Dairy Products	Special Treats
Bread	All fruits	Ice cream	Candy
Cereal	Beets	Milk	Chips
Corn	Carrots	Soy beverages	Chocolate
Crackers	Parsnips	Yogurt	Cookies
Legumes	Peas		Fruit juice
Lentils	Squash		Regular sodas
Pasta	Tomatoes		
Potatoes	Turnips		
Rice			
Roti, naan, injera			

Sugar

While carbohydrate is an important part of your child's diet, it is recommended to limit the amount obtained from free sugars. According to the World Health Organization's "Sugars Intake for Adults and Children" guidelines, the intake of free sugars — those that are added to food and beverages as well as those naturally present in honey, syrups, fruit juice and fruit concentrates — should be limited to no more than 10% of total energy intake.

Take, for example, a typical 9-year-old girl. Based on her estimated energy requirements, she should consume no more than 40 grams of free sugar per day. One teaspoon (5 mL) of sugar is about 4 grams. If you take a look at some of the examples below, you'll see that sugar adds up quite quickly!

- 1 can (12 oz/355 mL) regular soda: ~40 grams sugar (10 tsp/50 mL)
- 1 cup (250 mL) of fruit juice: ~25 grams sugar (6 tsp/30 mL)
- 1 cup (250 mL) of chocolate milk: ~25 grams sugar (6 tsp/ 30 mL)
- ½ cup (125 mL) canned tomato sauce: ~7 grams sugar (1.75 tsp/8.5 mL)
- 1 yogurt tube: ~7 grams sugar (1.75 tsp/8.6 mL)

Did You Know?

No Judgment

When talking about food, it is important to not attach judgment or shame. Just as when talking about blood glucose levels, do not use the words *good* and *bad* when referring to foods. Rather, try using the terms *everyday* and *sometimes* foods.

Fiber

Fiber is a type of carbohydrate that the body cannot digest. This means that it does not have a direct impact on your child's blood glucose. It is found in plant-based foods such as whole grains, vegetables, fruits and legumes. Fiber is an important part of your child's diet.

There are two types of fiber:

1. **Insoluble fiber:** This type of fiber can help you feel fuller for longer and prevent constipation. You can find insoluble fiber in whole grains, wheat bran, seeds and the skins of vegetables and fruits.

2. **Soluble fiber:** This type of fiber absorbs water and turns into a gel. This helps to lower cholesterol and prevent constipation. Soluble fiber can be found in oats, psyllium, apples, oranges, carrots and legumes.

Recommended Amount of Fiber Based on Age		
	Age	Adequate Intake (AI)
All children 8 and under	1–3 years old	19 g/day
	4–8 years old	25 g/day
Males	9–13 years old	31 g/day
	14–18 years old	38 g/day
Females	9–13 years old	26 g/day
	14–18 years old	26 g/day

Protein

Protein is critical for growth and to promote healing and tissue repair. Foods with protein contain many essential vitamins and minerals. They include:

- Meat, poultry, fish and shellfish
- Eggs
- Milk, yogurt, cheese and other dairy products
- Legumes (beans, chickpeas, lentils, peanuts, peanut butter, tofu)
- Nuts

With the exception of milk, yogurt, ice cream, nuts and legumes (which also contain carbohydrate), protein foods do not directly raise blood glucose levels. However, during periods of starvation or undernutrition, the body can break down protein into glucose.

Fat

Fat is an important part of a well-balanced diet. Fat provides energy and important building blocks for growth and development. Fat also helps the body absorb vitamins A, D, E and K. Examples of fat include:

- Oils, lard, shortening, margarine
- Dairy products such as butter, milk, cream and cheese
- Salad dressings
- Gravy
- Nuts and seeds
- Olives
- Coconut
- Avocado

There are three different types of fat:

1. **Unsaturated fat:** Unsaturated fats are liquid at room temperature. Eating these types of fat, instead of saturated and trans fats, helps to lower low-density lipoprotein (LDL) — the "bad" cholesterol.

    - Monounsaturated fat: found in olive and canola oils, nuts and avocados
    - Polyunsaturated fat: found in fatty fish, nuts, seeds and ground flax

2. **Saturated fat:** Saturated fats are solid at room temperature. Eating this type of fat can increase LDL cholesterol. Found in: animal products such as milk, cheese, butter and meat, as well as coconut and palm oils.

3. **Trans fat:** Trans fats are created by a process called hydrogenation, which changes the fat from liquid to solid at room temperature. This type of fat increases LDL cholesterol and also decreases high-density lipoprotein (good) cholesterol. Found in: some margarines and many commercially baked and fried foods, such as cookies, cakes and frozen foods.

Did You Know?
Financial Constraints

The food your child consumes has a big impact on their diabetes management, but some families may find it especially challenging to follow nutrition recommendations due to limited financial resources. If you are having difficulty affording food for you and your family, let your diabetes team know, as they may be able to offer tools and strategies to manage this challenge.

Did You Know?
Good and Bad Cholesterol

The terms *good* and *bad* have been widely applied to those types of cholesterol less or more likely, respectively, to contribute to cardiovascular risk. When planning your child's meals and snacks, focus on including unsaturated fats, limiting saturated fats and avoiding trans fats.

"Free" Foods

Foods that do not contain a significant amount of carbohydrate are sometimes referred to as "free foods." We typically do not match insulin to these types of foods, so your dietitian may advise you that these foods can be eaten outside of scheduled meal and snack times.

Here are some examples of free foods:

- Most vegetables, including: cucumbers, celery, broccoli, cauliflower, green beans, spinach, lettuce and kale
- Unbreaded meat, poultry, fish and shellfish
- Eggs
- Cheese
- Most dips and dressings
- Fats

It is important to remember that while these foods contain little to no carbohydrate, this does not mean they can be eaten in unlimited quantities. Meat and cheese have many nutritious properties but should be eaten in moderation, as they are also high in saturated fat and calories. When choosing free-food snacks, try choosing vegetables more often than the others.

> Meat and cheese have many nutritious properties but should be eaten in moderation, as they are also high in saturated fat and calories.

Drinks Count!

It's easy to forget that drinks can add extra carbohydrate and energy to your child's or teen's diet, without helping them feel full or contributing important nutrients. It may surprise you to learn that a fancy specialty coffee drink can add up to the same amount of carbohydrate and energy as a fast-food burger and fries! Or that a can of regular iced tea has the same amount of sugar as a cup (250 mL) of ice cream! The bigger the size and the fancier the drink (think added syrups and whipped cream), the more extra sugar and energy your child will be consuming.

Your best bet is to stick to water or milk most of the time, and limit sugar-sweetened beverages as much as possible. Rather than a regular soda or iced tea, try offering soda water with added lemon, cucumber or frozen berries. If your teen is ordering a specialty coffee drink, suggest they select the smallest size and ask for half-sweet, unsweetened or sugar-free syrup. And remember to check the nutrition information so that you can match the amount of carbohydrate with insulin.

Another surprise: One cup (~250 mL) of a regular soda (and not the ones with extra sugar to provide an energy boost) has about the same amount of sugar and energy as does the same amount of "unsweetened" orange juice!

Carbohydrate Counting

Now that you know which foods contain carbohydrate, it is time to start thinking about how much carbohydrate is in each of the foods your child or teen eats. Carbohydrate is measured in grams, and knowing the number of grams your child is consuming at a meal or snack will be important in order to properly match this against the appropriate dose of insulin.

In the beginning, it can be helpful to think of carbohydrate foods in terms of 15-gram portion sizes. Here are some examples of commonly eaten foods, listed in portion sizes that equal roughly 15 grams of carbohydrate:

- 1 slice of bread
- 1 medium apple
- 1 cup (250 mL) cow's milk
- ½ cup (125 mL) cooked pasta
- ½ cup (125 mL) fruit juice
- ¾ cup (175 mL) plain yogurt
- ⅓ cup (75 mL) cooked rice
- ½ medium potato
- ½ cup (125 mL) cooked lentils

Often parents will ask, "How much carbohydrate should my child or teen be eating?" While there are general recommendations based on age, it is important to take into account their appetite and activity level when determining carbohydrate targets. Your dietitian will ask you to complete food records in order to get a sense of your child's or teen's typical intake. As long as your child or teen is consuming a healthy, balanced diet and is growing and developing appropriately, there is no reason to change his or her typical carbohydrate intake.

How to Read a Nutrition Label

There is a lot of information found on a nutrition label. At first, it may seem overwhelming to try to make sense of all the numbers listed. Your child's dietitian can help you navigate the nutrition facts table and ingredient list. For the purpose of carbohydrate counting, there are only three things you must look for on the label.

1. Look at the serving size and compare it to the amount of food being eaten.
2. Look at the total amount of carbohydrate, which includes starch, sugars and fiber.
3. Look at the amount of fiber and subtract it from the total carbohydrate (because it does not raise blood glucose).

American Bread Label

Nutrition Facts

Serving Size 3 oz (2 slices)

Amount Per Serving

Calories 170	**Calories** from Fat 15

	% Daily Value
Total Fat 2.7 g	**4%**
Saturated Fat 0.5 g	**5%**
Trans Fat 0 g	
Cholesterol 0 mg	**0%**
Sodium 200 mg	**8%**
Total Carbohydrate 36 g	**12%**
Dietary Fiber 6 g	**24%**
Sugars 3 g	
Protein 8 g	

Vitamin A 1%	•	Calcium 2%
Vitamin C 0%	•	Iron 16%

* Percent Daily Values are based on a 2,000 calorie diet. Your Daily Values may be higher or lower depending on your calorie needs.

	Calories	2,000	2,500
Total Fat	Less than	65 g	80 g
Sat Fat	Less than	20 g	25 g
Cholesterol	Less than	300 mg	300 mg
Sodium	Less than	2,400 mg	2,400 mg
Total Carbohydrate		300 g	375 g
Dietary Fiber		25 g	30 g

Canadian Bread Label

Nutrition Facts

Per 90 g serving (2 slices)

Amount	% Daily Value
Calories 170	
Fat 2.7 g	4%
Saturated 0.5 g + Trans 0 g	5%
Cholesterol 0 mg	
Sodium 200 mg	8%
Carbohydrate 36 g	12%
Fibre 6 g	24%
Sugars 3 g	
Protein 8 g	

Vitamin A	1%	Vitamin C	0%
Calcium	2%	Iron	16%

At first, it may seem overwhelming to try to make sense of all the numbers listed. Your child's dietitian can help you navigate the nutrition facts table and ingredient list.

Using this example, here is how you would calculate the net carbohydrate: 36 grams – 6 grams = 30 grams. Two slices of this bread equals 30 grams of net carbohydrate. If your child was eating only one slice (half of the serving size), you would divide this number in two.

Did You Know?
Nutrition Scale

Another way to accurately estimate carbohydrate content is to use a nutrition scale. Using a database and the food's weight, a nutrition scale will display the nutrition information for that food. A scale is especially helpful for items where serving size is harder to estimate, like fruits and vegetables.

HOW TO: Handle Sweets and Treats

In many cases, the first question a child or teen will ask after diagnosis is, "Can I still eat [insert favorite food here]?" In short, *yes*, your child can still enjoy treats even after being diagnosed with type 1 diabetes. It is a common misconception that people with diabetes cannot eat sweets. However, it is important to consider the portion size and frequency of these special foods. Just as it is recommended to a child without diabetes, treats should be eaten in moderation. A general rule of thumb is to offer treats no more than once or twice a week.

Remember, treats should be enjoyed and savored — your child or teen should not feel guilty about eating these types of food. Consider enjoying treats together as a family. For example, a family walk to the ice cream shop can be a fun way to incorporate a treat into the diet of someone with diabetes.

Meal Planning Considerations for Different Insulin Regimens

The various insulin regimens are described in detail in chapter 4. Knowing what types of insulin your child or teen takes and how they act in the body will help you better understand the meal planning recommendations outlined below.

BID or TID Routine

This type of regimen requires consistency in timing and amount of carbohydrate. In these routines, insulin is matched to carbohydrate by consuming a consistent amount of carbohydrate and taking a consistent dose of insulin. As you develop and refine your carbohydrate counting skills, your dietitian will help to set target amounts of carbohydrate for each of your child's or teen's meals and snacks.

Carbohydrate targets should be based on appetite and nutrition requirements. When setting carbohydrate targets, a range of +/- 5 grams is typically used. This means that if your child's or teen's target for breakfast is 40 grams, anywhere between 35 and 45 grams would be considered in range.

Your child's satisfaction with the amount of food is important. The goal is for your child or teen to feel comfortably full (not stuffed!) at the end of each meal or snack. Meal plans will change as children grow.

Pro Tip

Pay attention when hunger increases or decreases, as this is a signal that carbohydrate targets and portion sizes should be reassessed.

MDI or Insulin Pump Routine

These methods of insulin administration allow for more flexibility in the timing and amount of carbohydrate. Rather than eating the same amount of carbohydrate and taking the same dose of insulin, an insulin-to-carbohydrate ratio can be used to vary these amounts from day to day.

While this routine is more flexible, it is still advised that your child or teen follows a routine and consumes healthy, balanced meals and snacks.

Example of Using a Carbohydrate Ratio

Ratio: 1 unit of fast-acting insulin for every 10 g (1 u:10 g)

Carbohydrate eaten at breakfast: 30 g
$30 \text{ g} \div 10 \text{ g} = 3$ units of fast-acting insulin to be given

Carbohydrate eaten at lunch: 60 g
$60 \text{ g} \div 10 \text{ g} = 6$ units of fast-acting insulin to be given

Did You Know?
Be Realistic

In many cases, it is neither practical nor realistic to set strict food amounts for a young child with diabetes. Rather, meal planning should focus on normal feeding, emphasizing healthy eating and creating a pleasant eating environment.

Meal Planning Considerations for Different Age Groups

The age of your child is an important factor when planning for the dietary management of their diabetes care. This is also something that will continue to change as your child grows and develops and has different food preferences, likely consumes larger quantities, and even eats in different settings, with potentially more variable timing around meals.

Under 5 Years Old

Young children experience fluctuations in appetite. The amount your child eats may vary widely from day to day. Young children may go through periods when they want to eat the same thing every day, followed by periods where they refuse to touch their previous favorites. This is normal. While these fluctuations are expected, they can make sticking to a meal plan challenging.

It is recommended that you learn about carbohydrate counting and aim for consistent amounts of carbohydrate. However, the target carbohydrate range will be wider for a young child than for older children. As mentioned previously, when a carbohydrate target is established, a range of +/- 5 grams is typically used. For a young child, it may be more realistic to set a range of +/- 10 grams. Even this wider range may not work for some children. Your dietitian will help set a plan that is individualized for your child.

The amount of time your child spends at the table will be dependent on their age. Young children may have the attention span to sit for only 10 minutes or so. Once your child has left the table, their mealtime is over and they should not be allowed to graze. Over time, your child will start to understand the meal schedule and know that food is offered during set times and not in between. Having routine, structured meal and snack times is advised for all children, whether or not they have type 1 diabetes.

You may find it stressful if you have given your child insulin and they are refusing to eat. Forcing a child to eat usually leaves both parent and child upset and frustrated. While you should not be a short-order cook, it is okay to offer a healthy alternative if your child is not eating the carbohydrate offered. You may consider offering fruit, unsweetened applesauce, yogurt, milk or a sandwich. Unless absolutely necessary, it is not recommended to replace meal or snack carbohydrate with treats or juice. This may lead to your child purposely refusing certain foods, because they know their favorite treat will be offered instead.

If your child has not consumed the target amount of carbohydrate at a meal or snack, watch carefully for a low blood glucose and treat it appropriately. If food refusal happens often, talk to your diabetes team. You may need to adjust the timing or amount of insulin.

School-Age

It is important for your child to aim for target carbohydrate amounts at each meal and snack, including when they are at school. To make it easier for your child to understand which food to eat at what time, try labeling their lunch and snack items. While meal and snack times can often be chaotic at school, it is important that teachers and other caregivers ensure that your child does not miss a meal or snack.

As your child gets older, it is good to start including them in the carbohydrate counting process. Try turning carbohydrate counting into a fun game. For example, at snack time, each family member can guess the amount of carbohydrate in the apples you are about to eat. If you have a nutrition scale, you can weigh the apples and see how close you were. Your child may also enjoy helping to portion out foods with measuring cups or helping to read the nutrition label.

Pro Tip

Mealtimes should be an enjoyable way to spend time as a family. Avoid distractions such as TV and handheld electronics during mealtimes.

Did You Know?
Open Discussions

It is not uncommon for children to trade foods when eating lunch at school. When discussing if your child may have eaten something outside of their meal plan, try not to blame or punish. Children may start hiding what they have eaten if they think they will get in trouble.

HOW TO: Involve Your Child in Cooking

It is beneficial to involve your child in age-appropriate meal preparation and cooking tasks. Not only will your child be more likely to eat foods they helped prepare, but you are also teaching them valuable life skills and spending quality time together. Here are some examples of what your child may be able to help with, based on age. Remember, children develop at different rates, so your child may be ready for certain tasks earlier or later than suggested.

Toddlers

- Helping scoop baking ingredients, like flour, into measuring cups
- Tearing lettuce into smaller pieces
- Kneading dough

6- to 7-Year-Olds

- Grating cheese
- Peeling vegetables
- Scooping batter into muffin cups

Kindergarten

- Mixing ingredients
- Using cookie cutters
- Cracking eggs

8- to 9-Year-Olds

- Using a can opener
- Beating eggs
- Cutting vegetables (with supervision)

Older children may be ready to start cooking more independently. However, it is always recommended that they be able to demonstrate safety precautions (like proper knife skills and turning pot handles in on the stove) and that there is an adult close by in the home.

It is also recommended to include your child in the meal planning process. When possible, involve your child in choosing grocery items — for example, allow them to pick the pepper or apple they think looks best. When planning meals, ask whether your child would prefer pasta or rice, or if they would like the potatoes roasted or mashed. If a child is given a choice, they are more likely to eat what they have chosen, compared to a meal where they have had no input.

Adolescents

Your teen may now have more extracurricular and social commitments than when they were younger, which can make eating regular, healthy, balanced meals and snacks more challenging. Factors such as peer pressure, sleeping in, skipping meals and attending parties have a huge impact on nutrition and blood glucose.

It is normal for teens to seek more independence, but it is also important that you continue to provide support around their nutrition management. Your teen may be capable of carbohydrate counting and calculating their insulin dose, but that does not always translate into these tasks getting done. Regular family meals together are a great way to continue to be involved with your child's nutrition and to spend valuable time together. You can gain insight into your child's carbohydrate counting skills and food choices at family meals, but remember that dinnertime conversations should not always focus on diabetes.

> Your teen may be capable of carbohydrate counting and calculating their insulin dose, but that does not always translate into these tasks getting done.

Glycemic Index

The glycemic index (GI) is a relative ranking of carbohydrate-containing foods based on how they impact the blood glucose. In other words, all carbohydrate foods are not created equal in terms of blood glucose effect. Foods are categorized as low, medium or high GI. Foods with a high GI ranking are digested and absorbed quickly, resulting in a higher and faster blood glucose spike. Conversely, foods with low GI rankings are digested and absorbed slowly and have a lower and slower blood glucose response.

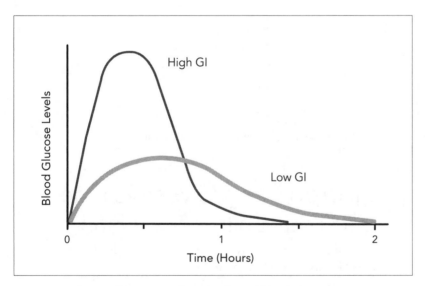

Source: www.glycemicindex.com/about.php

The effect of each food will also depend on the amount eaten. Foods with a low GI can help us to feel fuller for longer, making meals and snacks more satisfying. The GI is helpful information to consider as you plan your child's meals and snacks, but it does not replace carbohydrate counting or aiming for carbohydrate targets.

Examples of Low-, Medium- and High-GI Foods

	Low (<55)	Medium (56–69)	High (>70)
Breads	100% stone-ground whole wheat Pumpernickel Sourdough	Whole wheat Rye Pita	White bread, Kaiser roll or baguette
Cereals	All-Bran and All-Bran Buds Oat bran Special K	Oatmeal Puffed Wheat Shredded Wheat Cream of Wheat	Bran Flakes Corn Flakes Rice Krispies Cheerios
Grains	Barley Bulgar Quinoa Parboiled or converted rice Pasta/noodles Wild rice	Basmati rice Brown rice Couscous	Short-grain rice Rice millet Tapioca
Starchy vegetables	Sweet potato Yams Peas Corn on the cob	Potato (new, white)	Baked potato Mashed potato (white)
Fruit	Most fruit (apple, orange, grapefruit, kiwifruit, unripe banana, peach, plum, pear)	Raisins Ripe banana Cantaloupe Dates	Watermelon
Legumes	Lentils Chickpeas, black beans, kidney beans, split peas, soy beans, baked beans	Black bean soup Green pea soup	
Dairy products (and alternatives)	Milk Yogurt Soy milk	Ice cream	

Source: Adapted from GlycemicIndex.com, Sick Kids handout and Diabetes Canada resource

Incorporating Glycemic Index into Your Child's Meal Plan

A great rule of thumb is to aim to include at least one low-GI food at each meal and snack.

- Have pumpernickel, oat bran, stone-ground, and whole-grain breads instead of white bread.
- Prepare dishes with beans (such as kidney beans, black beans or pinto beans), chickpeas and lentils.
- Try choosing oatmeal instead of cold breakfast cereals (even Rice Krispies, Bran Flakes and Corn Flakes are high GI).

- Eat yams and sweet potatoes more often than white potatoes or french fries.

- Choose parboiled, long-grain or brown rice more often than instant or short-grain rice.

- Most vegetables, fruit and milk products have a low glycemic index — choose a variety of these foods every day.

- Continue to count the amount of carbohydrate in your child's meal plan to properly dose for the right amount of insulin.

Eating Out

For the first few weeks after diagnosis, you may be nervous about taking your child out for dinner. While home-cooked meals are encouraged, it is okay to eat at restaurants occasionally. Most chain restaurants have nutrition information available in-store and online.

If your child's meal is delayed and there is insulin peaking, try asking for breadsticks or a glass of milk while you wait. Make sure to incorporate these foods into your child's carbohydrate target for that meal. If your child is taking fast-acting insulin, wait until the meal arrives before administering the dose.

Friends and family who do not have experience with type 1 diabetes may be worried about what to feed your child. It may help to take the lead and invite friends and family over first so they can see that your child still eats the same foods as before. When eating at a friend's house, ask what foods they intend to serve and provide some guidance. Talk to your dietitian about ways you can adjust your child's meal and snack routine to accommodate meals served at different times or on special occasions.

Q & A

Q. Can my child still go to birthday parties and eat cake?

A. Yes, your child can still enjoy treats and fully participate in celebrations and special events. In fact, many children are so excited by the fun and games at a party that they end up consuming less food than usual, or being so active that they balance out the cake's impact on blood glucose. The key is to ensure that the adult in charge is aware of your child's diabetes and knows when and what your child should eat. And if the blood glucose is high that evening, note the reason in your child's logbook. Your child's diabetes team can help you plan for special events to ensure that diabetes does not get in the way of your child's participation and enjoyment.

As your family begins to make changes in the foods you purchase and consume, you may come across products or supplements that claim to help manage diabetes. It is important to let your team know if you are thinking of trying any natural health products, as some could be potentially harmful. Many of the claims made by these products are related to type 2 diabetes, and as you learned in chapter 6, type 1 and type 2 diabetes are very different. The mainstay of treatment for type 1 diabetes is insulin, and it cannot be replaced by any natural health product.

Q. What about fasting? Can children with diabetes participate in rituals of Ramadan or Yom Kippur?

A. Fasting can be dangerous for anyone who takes insulin. Generally, people with diabetes are exempt from these rituals, but you may wish to check with your religious authority. Older children and teenagers using an insulin pump or MDI insulin routine may be able to fast more safely. If your child is considering fasting, it is very important to speak with your diabetes team in advance, as insulin doses will need to be adjusted.

Q. I get tired of always being the "bad guy," always saying no when my 12-year-old asks for a treat other than at a meal or snack time. Any suggestions?

A. Some parents handle this situation by reversing the question: "Well, what do you think? Do you think you can have that treat and still keep your blood glucose balanced?" Most often, the child makes a sensible choice. Sometimes the question leads to creative problem-solving.

Q. Should my child start eating artificially sweetened products?

A. In general, your child does not require any specialty food products. Your child can continue to enjoy the same foods as the rest of the family. Some families choose to replace foods that have a very concentrated source of sugar, such as syrups and jams, with artificially sweetened versions.

You may notice that some products are sweetened with sugar alcohols, such as maltitol, sorbitol or xylitol. Sugar alcohols are only partly absorbed by the body and have little to no effect on blood glucose. It is wise to be aware of the amount of sugar alcohols consumed by your child, as amounts of over 10 grams per day may cause digestive upset.

Health Canada has approved the following sweeteners as safe if taken in amounts up to the Acceptable Daily Intake (ADI):

Safe Artificial Sweeteners

Sweetener	Common/ Brand Name	Forms & Uses	Other Things You Should Know
Acesulfame potassium (Ace-K)	Not available for purchase as a single ingredient	Added to packaged foods and beverages only by food manufacturers	Safe in pregnancy ADI = 15 mg/2.2 lb (1 kg) body weight per day (e.g., a 110-lb/50 kg person could have 750 mg of Ace-K per day). One can of diet soda contains about 42 mg of Ace-K.
Aspartame	Equal NutraSweet Private-label brand	Available in packets, tablets or granulated form Added to drinks, yogurts, cereals, low-calorie desserts, chewing gum and many other foods Flavor may change when heated	Safe in pregnancy ADI = 40 mg/2.2 lb (1 kg) body weight per day (e.g., a 110-lb/50 kg person could safely have 2000 mg of aspartame per day). One can of diet soda may contain up to 200 mg of aspartame.
Cyclamate	Sucaryl Sugar Twin Sweet'N Low Private-label brand	Available in packets, tablets, liquid and granulated form Not allowed to be added to packaged foods and beverages Flavor may change when heated	Safe in pregnancy (be cautious of exceeding ADI) ADI = 11 mg/2.2 lb (1 kg) body weight per day (e.g., a 110-lb/50 kg person could have 550 mg of cyclamate per day). One packet of Sugar Twin contains 264 mg of cyclamate.
Saccharin	Hermesetas	Available as tablets Not allowed to be added to packaged foods and beverages	Safe in pregnancy ADI = 5 mg/2.2 lb (1 kg) body weight per day (e.g., a 110-lb/50 kg person could have 250 mg of saccharin per day). One tablet of Hermesetas contains 12 mg of saccharin. Available only in pharmacies
Sucralose	Splenda	Available in packets or granulated form Added to packaged foods and beverages Can be used for cooking and baking	Safe in pregnancy ADI = 9 mg/2.2 lb (1 kg) body weight per day (e.g., a 110-lb/50 kg person could have 450 mg of sucralose per day). One packet of Splenda contains 12 mg of sucralose; 1 cup (250 mL) contains about 250 mg of sucralose.
Steviol glycosides	Stevia-based sweeteners such as: Stevia Truvia Krisda Pure Via	Table-top sweeteners Added to drinks, breakfast cereals, yogurt, fillings, gum, spreads, baked products and snack foods	Safe in pregnancy ADI = 4 mg/2.2 lb (1 kg) body weight per day (e.g., a 110-lb/50 kg person could have 200 mg of Stevia per day). A 30-g portion of breakfast cereal may contain 11 mg of steviol glycosides.

Source: www.diabetes.ca/diabetes-and-you/healthy-living-resources/diet-nutrition/sugar-sweeteners

Chapter 8

Adjusting to Life with Diabetes

From the day of diagnosis, diabetes has an immediate impact on the psychological, emotional and social functioning of the young person, as well as the family. In this chapter, we discuss how this changes through the years. As the child or teen matures, families will face emotional and social challenges that can cause barriers to the successful management of the diabetes. The good news is that most families navigate well through these times; if you run into trouble, the diabetes team is there to provide support and help to direct you to appropriate individuals trained to deal with these challenges: social workers, psychologists and other behavioral or mental health specialists.

Key Messages

- Most children and teens with diabetes and their families adapt well to living with this chronic condition.

- Families and diabetes team members need to keep an eye out for evidence of psychosocial stressors that can interfere with good diabetes control.

Dealing with the Diagnosis

The diagnosis of diabetes usually prompts a number of reactions in children or teens and parents. As discussed in chapter 1, most families experience a grieving period at first, with a variety of feelings that may include shock, denial, sadness, anxiety, fear, anger and guilt. Over time, most families do adjust and get on with life as they knew it, although always carrying the weight of the diabetes. You might find yourselves adapting and readapting, feeling some of these emotions not only at the time of diagnosis, but intermittently throughout you or your child's life with diabetes.

Critical transitions or changes in the family life cycle, including your child's developmental stage, also have the potential to prompt some of the feelings one initially experiences at diagnosis. However, you need to be aware that not all families go through the same grieving process at diagnosis, nor do all family members experience the same feelings at the same time. Grieving is a highly individual process.

Message of Reassurance

As you read this chapter, there may be the tendency to feel increasingly overburdened by the demands of diabetes care: How will our family cope? Will we be able to meet the demands of good diabetes control? Is diabetes going to take over our lives? And these feelings may escalate as you learn more about diabetes and the other things you need to consider because of their impact on its management.

Our extensive experience with many thousands of teens with diabetes is very reassuring: the vast majority incorporate diabetes into their daily routines and participate in activities just like their peers without diabetes. Children and teens living with diabetes don't miss more school or perform more poorly at school. They can participate in all school and extracurricular activities. They should have the same aspirations for their lives as they would had the diabetes not developed.

Emotional Responses

During the early stages after diagnosis, the support of the diabetes team, including the social worker and psychologist or behavioral specialist, is very important. These specialists can not only help stabilize the immediate medical condition, but also provide ongoing support, including anticipatory guidance, to the child and family. Don't be afraid to talk to your team about your emotional responses to the diabetes. This will help them to determine if you or your child is in need of support; it also provides an opportunity for them to review the facts about caring for a child or teen with diabetes, and to ensure that you are incorporating this knowledge into your daily lives without feeling overburdened.

> Don't be afraid to talk to your team about your emotional responses to the diabetes.

The emotions experienced by the child and family during this challenging time run the gamut from shock to guilt.

Shock or Denial

"This can't be true!" "I'm sure it's going to go away."

Often when we experience a crisis, our first reaction is shock. This is our body's way of cushioning the blow. It's natural to feel numb and, early on, parents often say the reality hasn't hit them yet. Others describe the feeling as a bad dream from which they keep hoping to wake up.

This feeling of shock is usually short-lived. Denial becomes unhealthy if it interferes with the family's ability to learn about their child's or teen's diabetes and carry out the day-to-day management tasks.

Anger and Resentment

"Why me?"

Young people can be angry about developing diabetes. They may hate the injections, blood checks and food restrictions, and feel their world has turned upside down. They may feel it just isn't fair that they have to deal with this disease and its demands.

Parents, too, can feel angry that this has happened, and helpless to change it. They may resent the extra responsibilities forced upon them. But anger can also empower parents in responding to and defending their child's needs.

Fear and Anxiety

"How will we ever cope?"

Confronted with diabetes and its implications, parents feel anxious about their child's health. Some worry about their ability to juggle the complex tasks required for good diabetes management, while others are more concerned about low blood glucose episodes. Some feel stressed about having to give injections or check blood glucose levels. Still others worry about their child's future health and wonder whether they will be able to manage alone in later years.

Some children fear injections or finger pricks in the beginning, and younger children, when they see their parents' distress, may even think they're going to die. However, their fear and anxiety often serve to focus the parents' attention on the needs of their children.

Sadness

"It feels like this is the end of the world." "I could never have imagined that one day we would wake up and our daughter would require insulin injections for the rest of her life."

When we grieve, we feel a sense of loss or a deep sadness. Parents can feel shattered by the knowledge that their child has to receive injections, do blood checks and follow a meal plan, and that these changes are likely permanent. Parents and children may mourn their old way of life. Children may be upset that they can't eat whatever and whenever they want to, or worry that it will affect their activities and friendships.

Did You Know?

Psychosocial Issues

There is no doubt that, when left unattended, psychosocial issues can become a major risk factor for persistent poor glucose control and increase the likelihood of earlier and more severe complications.

Parents may feel bad that they have to say no sometimes to even healthy food because it isn't the right time of day to eat.

Experiencing these emotions may help us begin to redefine our lives and put the pieces back together. Once people have expressed their sadness and sense of loss, they start to see the many parts of their lives, and the many hopes for the future, that don't have to change.

Guilt

"What did we do wrong?"

Parents often wonder if their child's diabetes is due to something they did, or blame themselves because diabetes runs in their family. Some feel guilty because they didn't notice the signs earlier. Children may feel they are burdening their parents. Some feel guilty, believing they must have done something wrong to cause the diabetes.

There is no reason to feel guilty: there is nothing anyone can do to cause or prevent type 1 diabetes.

Emotional Impact on Siblings

Diabetes impacts more than just the child with this condition; it also has a striking impact on the parents' interactions with their other children. As parents, you can become so focused on the child with diabetes that you may ignore a sibling's need for attention. This is not uncommon given the new demands that diabetes places on the family. The siblings without diabetes feel left out or abandoned when not actively included. The diabetes team can be a resource when it comes to distinguishing between healthy adaptation and fearful or anxious feelings that may interfere with the day-to-day functioning of the family.

Siblings go through the same emotions as other family members: guilt that their brother or sister has diabetes and they don't; fear that they, too, may get diabetes, or that their sibling may become really sick; anger that Mom or Dad stopped buying sugar-coated cereals or baking chocolate chip muffins; jealousy because their sibling seems to get all the attention.

It's a challenge, especially at the time of diagnosis, to balance everyone's needs. Brothers and sisters need to be given the opportunity to express their feelings and emotions, and to know that they are still loved. They should be encouraged to participate in the education program, both to involve them in the new family reality and to provide information that will allow them to feel safe and comfortable with their sibling with diabetes.

Pro Tip

Many parents find that spending "special time" alone with siblings who don't have diabetes eases the emotional impact on them.

Telling Friends

Childhood and adolescence are periods of frequent and intense social interaction. While parents are trying to figure out how to deal with daily diabetes management, young people are often more worried about how to incorporate this new reality into their lives. Plenty of questions arise: What do I tell my friends? How do I tell them? Will they treat me differently now that I have to take daily injections, check my blood glucose and eat my meals at specific times?

Just as each family has different ways of coping with diabetes in general, children and teens have different styles of telling their friends. With a little encouragement, most children will choose an open, matter-of-fact approach. Some make a presentation on diabetes to the class as part of show-and-tell. Others choose to share their experience and knowledge as part of a speech or science project. Most classmates are curious and full of admiration for a friend who is brave enough to do daily injections and finger pricks.

But not all children are comfortable with this approach. Some hesitate to discuss their diabetes with classmates they hardly know. Rather, they prefer to share the information

Pro Tip

Any time your child plans to spend time with a friend, make sure the caregiver is aware of the diabetes routines and knows the signs and appropriate treatment of a low blood glucose reaction.

only with school personnel and their closest friends, the ones they rely on for support.

One reason children want to avoid telling people is the fear of teasing or shunning. If teasing is an issue, children may need some special tips and support in handling the situation. Especially in the preteen and teen years, the priority is to fit in with peers to gain a sense of belonging and to not stand out as different.

We have heard from some young people that it's not only the negative attention they're trying to avoid but also the frequent questioning from teachers or peers as to how they're feeling. Young people who have experienced this situation report either feeling annoyed and/or ashamed about getting this much attention. Clearly a balance is needed — peers and teachers need to respond when there seems to be a real need for assistance while also respecting the young person's dignity and right to be treated like everyone else.

The family, the school and the diabetes team can all play a supportive role in helping the child talk to friends and deal with their varied reactions. Parents can speak to the friends' parents and help the child feel more self-confident. The school can explain to classmates that diabetes is not contagious, and that the child with diabetes is no different from other children and can continue to enjoy the same games and activities as before. Among the members of the diabetes team, the social worker or guidance counselor is usually best equipped to deal with these coping issues, recognizing children's varied backgrounds, personal experiences and family dynamics.

CASE HISTORY
"She Doesn't Want Anyone to Know..."

A frantic parent called one day to report that her 12-year-old daughter had experienced a severe hypoglycemic episode, with loss of consciousness and a probable seizure, while participating in her after-school competitive dance program. The dance teacher, Mom said, did not know what to do. She'd initially panicked, but did call 911, the emergency medical response service. Everything turned out well, but when carefully questioned, Mom said: "My daughter does not want anyone to know about her diabetes, so I had not informed the dance teacher about what needed to be done should my daughter start to have symptoms of hypoglycemia."

Living with Diabetes

Adjusting (coming to terms with or accepting the diabetes) takes time and patience for all family members. Given the pervasive nature of diabetes — it affects all aspects of daily living — it is essential that all members of the family be part of the diabetes support team. This means understanding, as far as they are capable (age, stage of development), the ins and outs of diabetes, and that they support and not undermine the treatment plan. Everyone may have to get up a bit earlier on weekdays to accommodate the new routine; children and teens may not be able to sleep in as late on weekends. Parents will need to plan meals in advance instead of acting spontaneously (at first, anyway) and will have to remember to pack extra food for the child when they leave the house. In the long run, though, these adjustments become second nature.

When the child with diabetes is very young, the overwhelming responsibility for care rests with the adults in their life — that is, parents or alternative caregivers. In two-parent families, one parent might play a predominant role, but it is essential for the other to support this and take over when needed. Whenever possible, both parents should be involved in all phases of the diabetes care routines. Feelings of resentment, fatigue and stress can build up if one parent is burdened with all the planning and responsibility. As parents, you should work together to prevent burnout by sharing the load and giving each other time away from diabetes duties. You need to plan time together, apart from your child or children, just as you did before. The child will also benefit from growing up in a household where diabetes responsibilities are shared evenly.

In single-parent families, it helps if a member of the extended family or a close friend can participate in the child's care from time to time, or provide relief by babysitting. Take steps, though, to ensure that babysitters and other caregivers know enough to look after a child with diabetes safely. Most diabetes teams will provide appropriate education for people participating in care at this level.

The challenge families face is to fit diabetes into their lifestyles, rather than letting it control their lives. This may require some creative problem-solving, often with help from the diabetes team. A strong support system of grandparents, aunts, uncles, siblings, friends and even support groups can do a lot to help you deal with the demands of diabetes, be it through practical or emotional support. Don't hesitate to ask for help from your diabetes team.

Pro Tip

If a spouse or partner is not available, it's important to look for outside emotional and practical supports from extended family or friends.

Did You Know?
Difficulty Adjusting

It will take some time to adapt to the "new normal" lifestyle of living with diabetes, as there are a lot of new things to get used to. However, if you find that within three months of diagnosis, you are continuing to feel overwhelmed and unsettled, it's best to reach out to your diabetes team with your concerns.

Indications of Successful Adjustment to Diabetes

- The child or teen is attending school regularly and participating in usual curricular and extracurricular activities.

- The child or teen has shared with friends the new diagnosis of diabetes. However, every child is unique, so it may take some a little more time to be open about their diabetes with their peers. For safety and psychological reasons, it is important that within a realistic period of time the child is able to share with friends their diagnosis of diabetes.

- The child or teen is cooperating appropriately in the performance of diabetes routines.

- The parents are able to leave the child with diabetes with an alternative caregiver (for example, babysitter) while they have some time for themselves.

- Blood glucose control is stable and meeting goals.

- The family is attending regular clinic visits and appropriately using the telephone hotline for emergencies only.

No doubt, the family that works together around diabetes care will see the fruits of their efforts in terms of better diabetes control/balance and less parent-child or parent-parent friction.

Attitudes and Beliefs

How families cope with diabetes depends to some extent on their attitudes and beliefs. Those who see it as a serious but manageable condition will cope better than those who remain overwhelmed, doubtful of their ability, or negative about the potential long-term consequences of the condition.

These attitudes and beliefs may be influenced by the family's prior experience with diabetes. Those who know someone having a difficult time, or experiencing serious complications, may feel very pessimistic about their own child's future. In this case, the diabetes team can help maintain perspective: science and technology have changed the outlook for people with type 1 diabetes, and there are positive steps you can take to decrease the chance of complications later in life.

At first, some parents view their child with diabetes as being sick or fragile. With a little time, education and experience, they soon learn that their child is still healthy.

Science and technology have changed the outlook for people with type 1 diabetes, and there are positive steps you can take to decrease the chance of complications later in life.

This is also an important message to give to your child or teen. Parents and caregivers have to resist the urge to be overly concerned and overprotective, as this may interfere with the child's normal development. Diabetes should not stop children and teens from doing all the things their friends do. It's just that extra planning and monitoring are needed to ensure their safety. This approach will go a long way in helping the child adjust to their diabetes as well as build their self-esteem.

CASE HISTORY
"She Goes Totally Ballistic"

A 15-year-old girl who has had type 1 diabetes for the past five years told us the following during her private time in the clinic: "My mom is great except for one thing when it comes to my diabetes: high blood glucoses! She asks me what my glucose level is every time I do a check. If it is higher than about 220 mg/dL (12 mmol/L), she goes totally ballistic. It's as if I've committed a serious crime."

Mom's response: "I am so worried about Angela's long-term health, what with all this talk about eye and kidney damage. So I hate to see high glucose readings. I know I overreact but I cannot help myself. I'm really doing it for her good."

Strategies for Adjustment

In addition to the usual and varied stresses that most families face, those living with diabetes must cope with additional demands. How can they ease the burden and adjust to the disease as smoothly as possible?

> Diabetes care can be complicated, and it's important not to think of outcomes as simply good or bad.

- **Learn as much as possible about diabetes.** Becoming an expert means you'll more likely be ready when a challenge arises.

- **Keep in regular contact with the diabetes team.** These health professionals are there to help with problem-solving. Sometimes a call to a team member can quickly solve a problem that seems impossible. Don't let a small problem grow.

- **Explore community and social supports.** Knowing other families who have a child or teen with diabetes, belonging to a parent support group or, for teens themselves, joining a diabetes youth group may lessen the tension by providing the opportunity to meet understanding peers.

- **Share the responsibility.** In two-parent families, find an appropriate balance of responsibilities and activities related to diabetes care. Single parents should try to find a support person who is willing to learn the basics about the child's diabetes routines and to provide necessary relief. With this backup in place, the child remains safe when the parent is not available.

- **Remember what worked before to relieve stress.** Fall back on familiar ways of coping that have worked in the past. This may involve taking time out, going for a walk, talking with a friend, listening to music or enjoying a vigorous physical workout. Self-care is not selfish!

- **Manage feelings — don't hide them.** Although it is often hard for parents to see their children upset, it is important to allow them to express painful feelings about having diabetes. This helps children feel understood and supported, and parents feel relieved knowing what the problem is. Solid communication builds trust and promotes problem-solving, important factors in healthy adjustment to a chronic disorder.

- **Use distractions.** For the small child, in particular, the actual performance of blood glucose checks and insulin injections may cause tension. Have the child hold a teddy bear during the injection, perform the finger pricks while the child watches television or have a sibling sit with the child while the routines are completed.

- **Try not to focus only on the diabetes.** Remember that children lead busy and active lives. Make an effort to focus on their schoolwork, their friends or their extracurricular activities. Get involved in these activities in a way that's consistent with your lifestyle, and demonstrate by your action and interest that diabetes is not your only shared activity.

- **Avoid black-and-white thinking.** Diabetes care can be complicated, and it's important not to think of outcomes as simply good or bad. Blood glucose and A1c levels should be thought of as high or low, not good or bad. Furthermore, diabetes care is not an all-or-nothing issue. Viewing temporary problems as slips, not failures, will make adapting easier.

- **Encourage positive behaviors.** Praising a child for their efforts can go a long way in building a sense of self-efficacy and self-esteem.

- **Problem-solve together.** Involve the young person in deciding what might be a viable solution.

Did You Know?
Diabetes Burnout

Experiencing diabetes burnout (see page 133) can be a normal part of living with diabetes. Do not feel you have to keep your feelings of fatigue, guilt, worry or being overwhelmed a secret from your family or your diabetes team. The team is available to support you through this difficult period.

Impact of Family Functionality on Diabetes Management

Just as diabetes has an impact on the family, the way a family functions has an impact on diabetes management. A healthy adjustment tends to be associated with the sharing of responsibilities, feelings of family togetherness, the ability to problem-solve, little conflict between family members, and consistent parenting. When there is overwhelming stress in the family, it's hard to think through problems and solve them effectively. As a result, diabetes care may be compromised.

A healthy attitude in the parents is key to helping children adjust; children take their cues from their parents and are sensitive to their feelings. When parents are consistent in their expectations and agree on the approach to diabetes management, the child is more likely to comply with routines. It also helps if parents are used to problem-solving and have developed coping strategies around stress in their own lives.

Settling into a Routine

In the weeks to months after diagnosis, the child or teen and their family will settle into their new routine. In some families this may mean very close attention to detail with very frequent monitoring and insulin adjustments. For others it may be a more relaxed approach.

The goals set for the family need to be clear (namely, target as near to normal blood glucose control as possible with as minimal a risk of severe hypoglycemia as possible); the approach, however, must be tailored to the needs of each family. In other words, the goals ought to be pretty **rigid** and well known to all, while the route to getting there can be much more **individualized**.

As you set your goals and start settling into a routine that works for your family, remember the three cornerstones of diabetes management:

- **Knowledge:** The more you know about diabetes, the better equipped you are to deal with unusual situations.

- **Motivation:** The more motivated you are about reaching targets, the less burdensome it can feel.

- **Execution:** The application of your knowledge and motivation to actually getting the job done.

As you set your goals and start settling into a routine that works for your family, remember the three cornerstones of diabetes management.

Keys to Success

There are a few keys to success when it comes to diabetes acceptance and management; these are easy for some families to incorporate into their daily lives, much less so for others.

1. Acknowledge the life-long nature of type 1 diabetes. This requires the support of the diabetes team to navigate the initial emotional responses to the diagnosis, as well as the stresses and strains that inevitably pop up along the way. It also requires not hiding the diabetes from people with whom the child or teen spends their time: school personnel, sports coaches and friends.

2. Learn all there is to know about taking care of the diabetes, and apply that knowledge very diligently.

3. Encourage the whole family to be part of the diabetes team, and, at home, to work as the child's or teen's core support group. This requires common goals that are transparent and achievable, and parental and sibling support for both the family member with diabetes and each other.

4. Thoughtfully avoid shame and blame. It's good to give praise when the goals of treatment are being met; it is, however, counterproductive to get upset when they are not. Preferably, try to analyze why things are going off course and correct them before they become serious problems.

Did You Know?

Striving for Perfection

Meeting the goals of diabetes care is not an easy task for most, if not all, families. Even the most dedicated families will not be able to achieve perfect control all of the time. However, it is important to remember that your best efforts do make a difference. If you feel discouraged or believe that your child's management plan isn't working, make sure to reach out to your diabetes team for the help you need.

Psychosocial Factors

The psychosocial factors that aid in successful diabetes management are:

- Family cohesion/inclusion, ability to resolve conflicts
- Expression of affect (feelings) and having empathy/ support
- Clear parental and child boundaries
- Good problem-solving ability

Did You Know?

Long-Term Outcomes

Recent research data suggest that the long-term outcomes for people with type 1 diabetes have been improving steadily over the past 50 years, with serious microvascular complications being reduced by more than half and a life expectancy that is approaching that of the nondiabetic population.

Preventing Complications

In the long run, the level of glucose control achieved and maintained will be the major predictor of the likelihood of the onset and/or progression of diabetes-related complications. Specifically, these complications are categorized into two groups:

- **Microvascular complications** affecting the small blood vessels of the body, especially in the kidneys (diabetic nephropathy), eyes (diabetic retinopathy) or nerves (diabetic neuropathy)
- **Macrovascular complications** affecting the large blood vessels of the heart (cardiovascular disease), brain (cerebrovascular disease) or limbs (peripheral vascular disease)

Unfortunately, the truth of the matter is that near normal glucose control is an enormously difficult goal to achieve and maintain, especially given the challenges of puberty, both biological and behavioral. Nonetheless, the best means of preventing these short-term complications is to monitor blood glucose frequently and keep a log of readings so that appropriate insulin dose adjustments can be made.

Keeping on Top of Things

In the clinic, we often overhear children with diabetes expressing feelings of frustration or discouragement:

- "I never get to take a day off from my diabetes."
- "Diabetes follows me wherever I go."
- "To stay in good shape, I need to think about my diabetes every 15 to 30 minutes."
- "There's certainly no entertainment value in this."
- "No matter how hard I work at my diabetes, I just do not seem to be able to reach the goals that have been set."

There is no doubt that type 1 diabetes is a relentless and never-ending condition. Although the vast majority of children and teens with diabetes feel very healthy most, if not all, of the time, they may well get bored of the constant need to stay on top of their condition. It's no wonder they sometimes feel like giving up. Yet, if they stop attending to their routines, things can slip quickly, resulting in high glucose levels and poor control, even diabetic ketoacidosis. Conversely, inattention to things like missed or delayed meals, or unanticipated exercise, can hasten hypoglycemic episodes.

Despite the seeming drudgery and the boredom that can come with attending to all the things that need to be done, remaining vigilant will certainly pay off in the long run in terms of better control and less risk of serious complications.

CASE HISTORY
"You're Just Too Lazy"

Mladen's dad always accompanied him to clinic. As Mladen got into his early teens, his A1c started to creep higher and higher. The doctor suggested that Mladen's parents should perhaps supervise or give his insulin injections and do his blood glucose for a while, in order to ensure that the testing was accurate and to prevent missed insulin injections. Dad became angry with Mladen. He said to him, "If you don't improve your control, your doctor is going to have to admit you to hospital. You're just too lazy and don't do anything other than play games on your phone." A father-son mudslinging match followed. When the temperature in the room had settled, the doctor asked Mladen to take a seat in the waiting room. She then gently but firmly asked Dad to never again use her or other members of the diabetes team as a threat.

Balancing Supervision with Independence

Dina is a 10-year-old girl who has had diabetes for four years. "It's her diabetes," says her mom each time they come to clinic. "I have two other children, a husband, a dog and a goldfish to take care of as well. Dina has got to take responsibility. After all, I won't always be there to take care of her."

Billy is now 8, having developed diabetes at the age of 2. His parents report: "We did everything for him, injections, blood glucose tests and much more. As he becomes older and is able to understand more, he wants to take care of his diabetes by himself. It has been very difficult for us to determine how and when to step back and let him take over his own care."

These two seemingly opposite scenarios demonstrate a few themes in diabetes management, which can be expressed as a series of questions:

- Whose diabetes is it?
- When should parents begin to let go, and how should they go about this?
- How will parents be able to judge whether they have acted appropriately?
- How will parents be able to prevent their anxieties from spilling out and affecting their child's ability to take over some, and eventually all, of the day-to-day responsibilities related to their diabetes?

Diabetes requires that both the young person and the parents acquire new skills and take on new tasks. These added responsibilities inevitably alter family relationships. With very young children, total responsibility for all aspects of their day-to-day care will fall directly to their parents or alternative caregivers. When not in the direct care of these individuals, young children must be in an environment in which there is an informed and identifiable adult to assume these responsibilities. However, as the child grows and matures, they will acquire increasing knowledge of diabetes, both by "living with it" and by understanding more information. There will be a slow and steady shift from completely parent-oriented care through stages of shared care to complete independence of the late adolescent and young adult in all aspects of diabetes management.

> New responsibilities should be added only as the child or teen demonstrates competence with those parts of the treatment plan for which they are already responsible.

The transfer of responsibility must not be too rapid. New responsibilities should be added only as the child or teen demonstrates competence with those parts of the treatment plan for which they are already responsible. The children who run into the most difficulty with their diabetes are those for whom parental support is either lacking or inconsistent.

Some health care providers mistakenly encourage families to give as much responsibility as possible to the child. After all, they argue, it's the child's diabetes and the child must become expert in its management. The best balance, however, requires that parents continue to support and encourage their children when it comes to achieving and maintaining the best possible level of glucose control. Parents obviously walk a thin line between giving too much responsibility too early and being overprotective.

Even when a young teen has been responsible for a good deal of diabetes care without much supervision, the parents will need to become more involved when the going gets tough, such as during periods of illness, stress at school or other emotional crises.

CASE HISTORY

Adult Supervision Required

We heard this cute story from a teacher who was doing playground duty for a preschool class. Since her spouse has had type 1 diabetes for many decades, she recognized what the 4-year-old girl off to the side of the playground was doing: checking her own blood glucose. She went over to talk to the child, who said that her mom had taught her how to prick her finger and do her glucose on her meter. The teacher asked her what her reading was. The little girl, who was reading her results in mmol/L, replied: "First there is a seven, then a dot, and after the dot, there is a six." The teacher thought, 7.6 mmol/L (136 mg/dL) — that's great. She said: "Anything else?" The girl said: "Oh yes, there is a one before the seven." So the reading was 17.6 mmol/L (nearly 320 mg/dL), not 7.6 (136 mg/dL)!

It seems as if the parental expectation of the 4-year-old was just too much. At that age, she would need support from a responsible adult in doing her glucose and then responding to it.

Diabetes Self-Management

Formal instruction in diabetes self-management must be appropriate to the child's developmental stage. While developmental stage and age are closely linked, not all children are ready to process information about their diabetes at the same time. Adults must watch carefully to be sure that the routines performed by the child are accurately done before slowly decreasing their level of supervision.

The best way to start is by ensuring they understand, in a developmentally appropriate way, why they are getting insulin injections or infusions, blood glucose tests, et cetera. The next step is to break down each task into its components and involve the child in these components, starting with the simplest and moving ahead as they demonstrate mastery of the previous step. The following box (page 132) is an example of the step-by-step approach to blood glucose testing.

Even when the child has learned the whole process well, the parents must ensure that the child continues to execute it well for a while before allowing self-management in the absence of the responsible adult. When control seems to be slipping (more variability in glucose test results, for example) or during a crisis such as an illness (cold, flu, gastroenteritis), closer parental control is once again required. Sometimes, parents may take over as children show some fatigue with the incessant demands of their diabetes.

> Adults must watch carefully to be sure that the routines performed by the child are accurately done before slowly decreasing their level of supervision.

Blood Glucose Testing, Step by Step

1. Lay out testing equipment: glucose meter, finger-pricking device, strips for meter.

2. Wash and dry hands to ensure no glucose on fingers.

3. Choose site for finger prick, rotating between fingers of both hands.

4. Place glucose strip in meter.

5. Pick appropriate finger.

6. Prick finger in appropriate spot with finger-pricking device.

7. Milk drop from finger prick.

8. Place blood on strip in the meter.

9. Get readout from meter and record in appropriate place.

Did You Know?

Laying the Foundations

The day will come when the teen with diabetes is no longer living under the family roof. This transition can be traumatic for both child and parent. No longer will you be able to monitor your teen's daily log of insulin doses and glucose readings. Nor will you be around to pick up on your teen's trademark symptoms of an insulin reaction. What is the solution? Start laying the foundations for independence early on. Encourage and support your child's age-appropriate involvement in their own diabetes care.

We used to expect children with diabetes to have achieved injection independence by 8 or 9 years of age. More recently, this expectation has been relaxed, and many do not achieve this stage before 10 to 12 years. If we wait too long, it sometimes takes a longer period of teaching and observation before these parts of the routines are incorporated into the child's or teen's daily expectations. Positive reinforcement is helpful at all stages once mastery has been achieved and demonstrated.

It remains necessary for parents or other caregivers to discuss testing results with their child or teen, and to reinforce the need for the child to seek assistance when challenged. Given the relentless nature of diabetes, and the often-negative parental response to high test results, it is not so unusual for some teens to miss their insulin injections and/or blood tests or report misleading readings to their parents. The physician/diabetes team checkup that takes place every three months gives time for this possibility to be explored in a nonjudgmental manner. Noncompliance with treatment routines is commonplace in teens with diabetes. The members of the health care team need to keep these ideas high on their radar and nip them in the bud as soon as they are detected.

Does Diabetes Care Add Up?

We like to think of diabetes care being governed by the "100% Rule" — that is, the input from the parents and/or other adults plus that of the child or teen with diabetes should always add up to 100%, which is the amount of care required to maintain excellent metabolic control and avoid hypoglycemia and ketoacidosis.

If the parents relinquish their role more rapidly than the child or teen accepts responsibility, then, at a critical stage, the sum is less than 100%, and inevitably things begin to be neglected and less than optimal care is provided.

If the parents hang on to their roles for too long, after the child or teen had begun to take on more and more responsibility, then the sum is greater than 100%, and the stage is set for difficulties over too much attention being paid. The ensuing battles over turf can have negative effects on the desired outcomes.

Diabetes Burnout

Diabetes burnout is an often-used term that remains ill-defined. What is meant is that the individual with diabetes and/or their parents get tired and frustrated with having to perform all of their diabetes routines day in and day out and want to throw in the towel for a while. Burnout can be characterized by the individual disregarding their blood glucose levels. They may also miss doctor appointments, forget or avoid taking insulin injections or other diabetic medication, or develop unhealthy eating habits. The A1c tends to rise and there may even be one or more episodes of diabetic ketoacidosis. At times like this, a responsible adult or adults need to step in and take charge until the situation can be rectified.

A person experiencing a burnout who adopts self-destructive behavior may subsequently suffer from fatigue and/or hypoglycemic episodes. Burnout is also often accompanied by psychological stress, anxiety, depression, anger, resentment, shame, guilt and helplessness.

There are a number of steps that can be taken to help avoid or diminish feelings of diabetes burnout:

- Manage your expectations: perfectionism is not the goal!
- Communicate empathy to your child or teen.
- Get support.
- Consider your values and your goals.
- Promote effective communication with your child and health care team.

Did You Know?
Parent Burnout

Diabetes burnout can also occur in a caring parent who becomes frustrated with the inability to meet targets despite best efforts.

- Include rewards for your child as well as for yourself.
- Engage in self-care and self-compassion.
- Become aware of your own emotional reactions that might be causing you and/or your family undue stress.

Research Spotlight

The Burden of Diabetes

Throughout this book we have emphasized that diabetes is a serious condition and, as such, deserves to be taken seriously. Some years ago, this fact was emphasized in a study that evaluated the impact of disease in families of teens with either type 1 diabetes or cancer. In the first five years after diagnosis, parents of children with cancer expressed more negative feelings and worries than those whose child had diabetes. Over time, with the cancer in remission, there was a crossover of findings: at 10 and 15 years, the parents of children with diabetes now expressed significantly more stress.

In another study, teens with diabetes showed increasing signs of the burden of their diabetes over time, while their health care professionals and parents reported some decline in burden as the teens supposedly progressed to self-management. This study suggests a lack of connection between the teen with diabetes and both their health care providers and parents. Our interpretation is that the relaxation of parental support likely leaves some teens at risk for stress.

Parenting a Child with Diabetes

One of the main focuses of this book relates to parenting a child or teen with type 1 diabetes. Many of the stories presented are about parent-child or parent-teen interactions and conflicts; almost all involve parental concerns. And, after all, our approach to caring for diabetes in children and teens is family-centered.

The case histories scattered throughout this chapter are full of lessons:

1. Recognize that blood glucose levels, while needing to be kept in check, do not define whether you have a good or bad kid, nor whether you are a good or bad parent (the words *good* and *bad* are used here in an intentionally judgmental way in order to illustrate the extremes of emotions or responses).

2. Support your child's desire for involvement in their own care, but be sure the handover of responsibility is a slow and carefully monitored process: the younger the child, the slower the transfer.

3. Stay vigilant. Even when your child or teen takes over their diabetes care in a responsible manner, it is still important to check in from time to time. Just asking for a verbal report is insufficient: checking the meter or pump memory is much more revealing.

4. Don't hesitate to get involved again. During periods of illness or heavy exercise, it is important for parents to take back some of the responsibility.

5. Avoid extreme reactions. If you find out directly or are informed by your diabetes team that your child or teen has been fudging their blood glucose readings or missing insulin injections, avoid getting angry and shaming them. They're not the first nor will they be the last to do this. Never forget that it is tough work looking after their diabetes. Two things work well: first, take back the responsibility for a while at least; that is, do the blood glucose tests and give the insulin injections. Second, ensure that you are seen as supporting their efforts, not as the enemy.

6. Don't use others to do your "dirty work." In the one case history, the dad threatened that his son's diabetes physician would mete out punishment for poor results — namely by admitting him to the hospital if he didn't shape up. Hospital admission is rarely the solution to a diabetes management issue, given that it is such an artificial situation compared to what goes on at home. Best to try to resolve the problems within the context of the son's daily life.

Principles of Parenting

What are the keys to good parenting? Many books have been written about what makes a good parent, but one thing is perfectly clear: parenting is not a one-style-fits-all experience. Our parenting styles will be influenced by many factors, both societal and individual.

Here are a few principles to live by, with a diabetes bent added in. Remember that what you do as a parent matters (even when you're ready to tear your hair out!)!

1. Good parenting requires **presence** — even more so with a younger child. Presence has two connotations. The first is physical presence: the act of simply being

CASE HISTORY

"Fudging" the Results

At a recent clinic visit, Devon, age 11, with diabetes since infancy, came with his mom, who brought his blood glucose logbook in which he had dutifully recorded all of his readings, never less than three per day and none above 180 mg/dL (10 mmol/L). Yet when his diabetes nurse downloaded his meter, there were very few recorded blood glucoses and none that matched with those in the logbook. Not surprisingly, Devon's A1c, 7.8% just before he went to summer diabetes camp for two weeks, had risen to 10.2% early in the new school year.

Mom was dumbfounded. What had changed? Nothing, Mom said. But more careful exploration revealed that Devon had returned from summer camp very proud of his ability to perform blood glucose testing and insulin injections, and, like some of his friends at camp, wanted his parents to leave him to do these unsupervised. His mom and dad had been reluctant at first, but over a couple of weeks, Devon won them over by exhibiting his ability to perform these tasks. His parents relented.

Initially, Mom did not believe us when we said that Devon had been "fudging" his blood glucose results and likely missing a significant number of insulin injections. When Devon admitted to this, Mom started to get very angry with him. "Whoa!" his diabetes doctor said. "Let's put this in perspective before war breaks out."

> If boundaries are reasonable and rational, they will help to cultivate respect and discipline. If they are inconsistent or erratic, the child or teen will become confused and often anxious.

there allows a developing young child to have a rallying point from which they can venture out and to which they can return. The second is emotional presence — meaning that when Mom, Dad or a primary caregiver is present, that person focuses positively on the child or teen in all their dimensions; this is often referred to as "quality time." The critical factor here is tuning in to the child's emotional state and providing emotion coaching and problem-solving as needed. Children also learn by watching their parents' behavior — and, hopefully, we all learn through our mistakes.

2. Setting consistent **boundaries** provides necessary structure and security for the developing child. The boundaries will change as the child grows up and shows evidence of maturing behavior. If these boundaries are reasonable and rational, they will help to cultivate respect and discipline. If they are inconsistent or erratic, the child or teen will become confused and often anxious. In a two-parent family, partnering between spouses is

important in being consistent. Discuss your family "rules" with your children and, as they mature, be sure to adapt them to the young emerging teen.

3. **Encouragement** on a regular basis is needed for the development of a positive self-image. Encouragement is different from praise for a job well done. Encouragement allows the child or teen to test their capabilities beyond the commonplace. When a chronic disease such as diabetes intrudes, it is far too easy to focus only on the negative — for example, high glucose levels and missed injections — and overlook the many other things the child or teen is doing. It is important to be aware of the positive and to encourage it whenever possible.

4. **Focus** on things that are important, but ensure that you do not only focus on the diabetes. All children are different, and parents need to adapt to fit their child. An extension of this principle is that parents should "choose their battles" with their children carefully. It's important to use discretion in deciding when to take on either an observer role or director role with your child: a messy room may be irksome but it's not worth daily arguments, while smoking is worth every effort to prevent or stop.

5. **Avoid harsh discipline:** Physical punishment and verbal abuse are demeaning to both parent and teen.

6. Treat your child with **respect**; only then can you expect respect from our child. Let your child act their age: don't expect too much too soon.

7. **Talk** to your child in a way that will help them listen, and listen to your child so they will continue to talk!

Parenting is a huge responsibility, and mostly a wonderful experience. You will know you need help if it seems as if you are *always*:

- Arguing with your child or teen or your spouse
- Breaking up arguments between siblings
- Constantly nagging your child or teen to do something, be it homework or diabetes routines
- Feeling unhappy about something (report cards, blood glucose levels, A1c)
- Resorting to either threats or bribes (for example, a dollar for every glucose test in the target range, or the threat of hospital admission if diabetes control deteriorates further)
- Feeling angry

Did You Know?
Make Mealtime Family Time

Try not to let the diabetes control the family agenda. Mealtime ought to be a time for family interaction around a whole host of topics, not just diabetes. We suggest that families try to sit down together for at least one meal each day, likely supper. Cell phones, tablets and other devices should be set aside to allow discussion of the day's activities and planning for the next day or days ahead.

Testing the limits and pushing back are features of normal adolescent development. The presence of diabetes merely raises the stakes.

If either parent or child feels this way, then something is amiss; attunement has been lost, at least temporarily.

It is good to remember that no single person is always right, making the other always wrong. There ought to be a middle ground, and that often needs to be negotiated. Testing the limits and pushing back are features of normal adolescent development. The presence of diabetes merely raises the stakes.

Financial Concerns

The ongoing cost of diabetes supplies can be a concern. The child or teen requires insulin; insulin administration devices; blood glucose monitoring equipment (meters and strips); urine test strips; glucagon emergency kits; and glucose tablets for low glucose reactions. Clearly, diabetes is expensive: for example, in both the United States and Canada, blood glucose test strips cost eighty cents to a dollar each. For someone checking blood glucose levels four or more times a day, this can add up to a considerable amount of money every year, for the strips alone.

Most extended health or private drug plans cover the cost of most diabetes supplies. For those who have no coverage and cannot afford these supplies, federal or state/provincial plans may help alleviate the burden. Volunteer agencies may also provide financial support. If you don't have private insurance and aren't eligible for government plans, these expenses should, at the very least, be eligible for a medical expense tax credit. If you're in this position, ask your diabetes team about agencies, resources and strategies that may help ease the financial load.

Q & A

Q. Our daughter does well in school but often complains of headaches or stomach cramps due to anxiety about going to school in the morning. What does this mean?

A. Your daughter may be experiencing school avoidance, which occurs commonly in children with a chronic condition such as diabetes. There are many reasons why children may become anxious. In a child with diabetes, the avoidance may have to do with being teased or with fear of having a low glucose episode while at school. Take time to explore your daughter's anxieties about school and diabetes, and seek help from your diabetes team. Ensure that she misses as little school as possible.

Q. People keep telling me I should join a diabetes support group, but I'm not sure if they're for me. What are they all about?

A. Support groups can be invaluable sources of information and advice and, in many cases, new friendships. Your diabetes team or local American Diabetes Association or Diabetes Canada (previously Canadian Diabetes Association) branch can provide names of group leaders. As well, many support groups form online and through social media sites. If there is no support group that meets your needs, you may want to start your own. Support groups meet on a regular basis — some follow formal agendas while others are casual social gatherings. There is little, if any, cost involved, and you're not obligated to attend every meeting. They may be a good place to find babysitters.

Some people resist support groups because they don't like the idea of identifying themselves as "afflicted." But in some ways, support groups free you from this label because everyone there knows the road you are traveling. You don't have to explain the biology and psychology of diabetes to get to the point of your problem. Sharing experiences provides a way to learn more about diabetes and to feel more secure about your effectiveness in dealing with it.

Q. My 9-year-old learned to give his own insulin injection at camp last summer and continued to do it regularly for the month after camp. But now he's lost interest and doesn't want to do it anymore. Should we insist that he carry on?

A. No. It's appropriate for you to take most of the responsibility for injections right now. He'll do it again when he's motivated. If he wants to go on a sleepover, he'll have to show you, a little while in advance, that he can safely manage this task.

Another tactic is to pull out a calendar and plan, together, a few days when he's going to give his shot with your supervision. This will maintain his confidence level.

Q. Every time Jack's grandparents come to visit, they shower him with chocolate and candy. How can we make them see this is harmful?

A. It's natural for grandparents to want to give gifts to their grandchildren. You may want to encourage them to pamper Jack in other ways, such as with trips to the movies, or snacks like popcorn. When the gifts are food, help Jack accept them graciously, and then help him work the treat into his meal plan.

Q. Will we ever take a vacation alone again?

A. It may take a while before you feel comfortable enough with your child's diabetes care to leave someone else in charge. But sooner or later you will. You can ease the anxiety by starting off gradually, with a short trip a couple of hours' drive away (you'll feel better knowing you can return home quickly), rather than a two-week vacation in South America. If you know, for example, that you have a weeklong business trip you can't miss, you can prepare yourself in advance by spending a night with friends or relatives.

Giving a sitter this kind of "dry run" may also alleviate their concerns, as well as the concerns of your child. Give your sitter and any siblings the telephone numbers of your diabetes health care team (and alert the team that they may be called by someone other than yourself). Provide relevant reading material and create a diabetes care instruction sheet specific to your child.

> Ease the anxiety by starting off gradually, with a short trip a couple of hours' drive away.

Chapter 9

Growth and Development

Each age and stage of life presents a different set of challenges relating to both physical and emotional growth and development. A chronic condition like diabetes often brings additional challenges. It seems that as soon as the family has found ways to negotiate their way through one stage of development, it's time to transition to the next stage. For example, parenting a school-age child with diabetes can be much different from parenting an infant or toddler. Likewise, being a teenager with diabetes is different from being 9 or 10 and living with diabetes. And as teenagers reach adulthood, they are faced with new issues that further affect their diabetes care.

> The best predictor of future behavior is past behavior: a child whose course has been relatively smooth throughout early childhood is quite likely to negotiate adolescence successfully.

Key Messages

- Different ages and stages of maturation bring different challenges with respect to diabetes care.

- Transition to self-management should be a slow, monitored process during which the parents relinquish responsibility only when their child has demonstrated competence with the routine.

- Parental involvement, with appropriate supervision, is an essential component of excellent diabetes care.

The family and the diabetes team can help smooth the road to adulthood by promoting a strong sense of identity and self-worth in the growing child. The best predictor of future behavior is past behavior: a child whose course has been relatively smooth throughout early childhood is quite likely to negotiate adolescence successfully. Also, families that provide age-appropriate support and guidance will no doubt have less disruption to deal with during the teen years. This means that you must go through a parallel process of development in relation to the development of your child or teen with diabetes.

In this chapter, we address the challenges of the main ages and stages of development — infant, toddler and preschooler; school-age; and adolescent — as well as the major transitions that occur between them (for example, going to school, increasing independence and self-care, and more).

Infants, Toddlers and Preschoolers

Type 1 diabetes is less common in preschoolers than in older children and adolescents: less than 1% of type 1 diabetes is diagnosed in the first year of life, and less than 10% before the age of 5. However, in recent years, there has been a trend toward diagnosis of type 1 diabetes at younger ages.

Because diabetes is less common in this age group and because the symptoms are often confused with other minor illnesses, the diagnosis is often missed until the baby or young child is very sick, and often in severe diabetic ketoacidosis. Once diabetes is diagnosed, however, the situation can be corrected quickly and long-term management can begin.

Developmental milestones and patterns affect the very young child's perception of the world. Normal infants and toddlers generally:

- Determine thoughts by what they see and hear.
- Begin to develop a sense of themselves, first by acquiring a trust in their environment as infants, and then by testing this environment in the next few years ("attachment").
- Enhance their knowledge of the world around them through constant exploration, language development and inquiry ("Why this? Why that? Why the other thing?").
- Begin to become more curious and self-directed, choosing some activities and rejecting others.

Diabetes care in children under 5 involves a balance between what might be considered ideal — close to normal blood glucose readings — and what is safe and practical. The target range for some of these young children may need to be a little higher than that for older children and teens with type 1 diabetes, at least to start (for example, before-meal glucoses of 110 to 220 mg/dL or 6 to 12 mmol/L).

In infants and toddlers, control that is too tight can be especially risky, as they cannot yet recognize the symptoms of low blood glucose. Similarly, it's important to avoid marked elevations in the blood glucose, which may lead to changes in mood and concentration.

Did You Know?

Anticipatory Guidance

Transitions are best dealt with by providing anticipatory guidance — that is, offering your child or teen an understanding of what to expect during the next phase/stage and how to prepare for some of these contingencies.

Very young children often have fluctuating appetites. They don't always eat the same amount of food from day to day. If blood glucose levels before meals are allowed to go slightly higher than those expected for older children, the infant or toddler is more likely to remain safe even during periods of food refusal or picky eating. Parents will be less worried and frustrated, and mealtime will be more pleasant.

As children grow, they become more predictable in their eating and more able to recognize and describe their low blood glucose reactions. At that time, blood glucose targets also change.

Pro Tip

Repeated episodes of severe hyper- or hypoglycemia in young children may lead to mild intellectual or learning impairment later in life.

Signs of a Healthy Infant or Toddler with Diabetes

- Normal growth and weight gain

- Meeting developmental milestones, such as rolling over, sitting up, crawling, standing, walking and talking

- No signs of high blood glucose levels; good energy; not overly wet (diapers) or unusually thirsty

- Few mild low blood glucose reactions, and no severe reactions

- No ketones in the urine

- Blood glucose readings that are not consistently too low or too high for long periods of time

- A happy and secure attitude in the child

Impact of Diabetes on an Infant, Toddler or Preschooler

Young children with type 1 diabetes progress through the same stages of development as their friends without diabetes. Nevertheless, the routines and tasks needed for good diabetes care may influence and sometimes interfere with this development. All parents of young children with diabetes worry about the effects of diabetes on their child's growth as an individual, and how they will cope with the condition as they grow older.

Diabetes care in children under 5 involves a balance between what might be considered ideal — close to normal blood glucose readings — and what is safe and practical.

Try to be quick, calm and reassuring when carrying out routines.

Specific areas of concern include:

- The young child's inability to express symptoms of hypoglycemia (for example, is the toddler having a low blood glucose or a temper tantrum?)
- Dealing with their own and their child's anxiety about the pricks and injections
- Developing a structured but flexible treatment plan that does not interfere with the child's normal daily activities, including naps
- Providing meals and snacks on time and in consistent amounts (toddlers with picky appetites can cause stress at mealtimes)

Try to balance your child's need for support and protection against the risk of overprotection and exclusion from age-appropriate activities.

Coping with Diabetes in a Young Child

- Try to adopt a matter-of-fact approach to insulin injections, finger pricks and mealtimes. Young children quickly pick up on their parents' anxieties and use them to manipulate their environment. Try to be quick, calm and reassuring when carrying out routines. Do not get angry with your child (sometimes easier said than done!). Reduce your child's fears by preparing the insulin or blood testing equipment in another room before involving the child. When it's over, give the child a big hug and a kiss.

- Share responsibility for the routines wherever possible. This prevents the toddler from playing one caregiver off against the other. In single-parent families, have a friend or family member participate in the diabetes routines on a regular basis. The parent, the toddler and the support person can remain confident that the child will be safe in the parent's absence.

- Acknowledge your child's feelings and provide reassurance, but don't delay needles or finger pricks until the child is "ready." Consider using distractions such as toys, songs or television.

- Try to allow your child some control over the routine if they wish — for example, choosing the finger for the next prick.

- For the really picky eater, set limits on the time allowed for meals and snacks. Don't sit for hours fighting over each morsel of food. The child always wins.

CASE HISTORY
Food Refusal

Tommy is 2½ and doing quite well with his diabetes routines. His parents, Heather and Marc, are sharing responsibility for his blood glucose checks and insulin injections. Heather gives the morning shot and Marc does the second one, before the evening meal. Tommy's 4-year-old brother, Tyler, is usually asleep during Tommy's morning routine — which suits Heather just fine — but Tyler likes to help his dad with the evening blood glucose check and insulin shot, leaving Heather free to get dinner on the table. Meal and snack times are consistent. Both boys enjoy settling in for their morning snack just as their favorite television program starts at 10 a.m. Afternoon snack works equally well, following Tommy's nap, at 3 p.m. The only problem for Heather comes when Tommy sleeps past 3 p.m. She hates to wake him, figuring he must need his sleep, but how long can she safely let him nap? Unlike children without diabetes, he can't nap right through his snack time. She decides, with the help of her diabetes team, that an extra half-hour is the limit.

Lately, Tommy has been refusing food, especially at mealtimes. Worried about lows, Heather and Marc have been pleading, coaxing and even preparing two or three food choices, but in the end, Tommy holds out for apple juice. After discussion with the diabetes team, Heather and Marc decide to reduce the insulin dose a little and raise targets to allow for food refusal, and to limit mealtime to a maximum of 25 minutes. They also plan to resist, if possible, replacing the meal with apple juice alone. Food refusal is a temporary stage many toddlers go through. As Tommy's appetite becomes more predictable, Heather and Marc will have to increase his insulin and reset his blood glucose targets.

School-Age Children

Starting school is an exciting and potentially challenging time for both children and parents. Children will now spend a major part of their day outside of the home and away from the parents' watchful eyes. But it is not until late childhood or early adolescence that a child should be expected to understand diabetes treatment fully and be able to integrate all its important concepts, such as the timing and amounts of insulin injections, blood glucose checks and consistency in eating habits.

Impact of Diabetes on a School-Age Child

During the school-age years, parents usually continue to be the predominant caregivers, but they are more frequently required to share expertise not only with the child but also with other responsible people such as teachers, sports coaches, babysitters and daycare staff.

School-age children with diabetes may see themselves as different from their peers, which can lead to considerable distress. Classmates may tease them about their needles and finger pricks. Be sure your child has an appropriate understanding of diabetes, but encourage them to participate in school and other activities in the same way other children do. Naturally, planning is required, but being excluded from these activities can be detrimental to the child's self-image.

Be sure your child has an appropriate understanding of diabetes, but encourage them to participate in school and other activities in the same way other children do.

Coping with Diabetes in a School-Age Child

- Remain actively involved in all aspects of your child's diabetes care throughout childhood. However, the level and type of your involvement will change as the child participates more and more in the routines. Ongoing parental involvement in a supportive and nonjudgmental manner will help the child to overcome hurdles along the way.

- Be prepared for the occasional slipup. As children assume more responsibility, they make mistakes — eating a little more, skipping a snack, recording a false blood glucose reading, perhaps even missing an injection. These lapses

CASE HISTORY

Preparing for a School Trip

Susan is 10 years old and has had diabetes since age 4. Her parents take most of the responsibility for her diabetes care, but Susan does help out. She has been able to do her own finger pricks and blood checks for a couple of years now, but she must be reminded when to do them. Her parents record the results. Susan is pretty good at choosing the right kinds and amounts of food at mealtimes and snack times. She knows what it feels like to be low, and she knows what to do: take three dextrose tablets.

She hasn't yet mastered her insulin injection; she just hasn't been interested, and her parents have been willing to stay in charge. But Susan is in fifth grade now, and her class will be going to an outdoor education camp for three days. Susan is determined to go too. Her parents are anxious and want to say no — but instead, knowing they have several months to prepare, they sit down with Susan and their diabetes nurse and come up with a plan that will prepare the family and the teacher for this adventure.

Because there may not be an adult on the school trip who can prepare and inject insulin safely, Susan's parents agree to work with her over the next few months to ensure that she is confident and competent with insulin injections by the time she's ready to go.

Susan is already able to do her blood glucose and ketone checks, so the next step is for her to begin entering results in the logbook for practice one week a month. Susan thinks this is a good idea.

Because she already makes good decisions about food choices every day, Susan's parents will begin to involve her in planning for extra activity with extra food.

Finally, Susan's mother will contact those at the school in charge of organizing the outdoor camp to find out about adult supervision, the program of activity, the meal schedule and opportunities for communication between Susan and her parents during camp. She will also organize an education session with the adult taking primary responsibility for Susan at camp. This person must remind Susan about testing and insulin injection times, supervise these routines, and, if necessary, help her respond to low blood glucose or get in touch with her family. These are not unrealistic expectations of an adult supervisor of a grade five student.

are a normal part of growing up. Expect them and watch for them so you can deal with them before there are any serious consequences. But remember that these lapses are not a sign of failure. Rather, they provide an opportunity to talk about diabetes and its challenges, and to open the door to creative problem-solving.

- Establish routines, such as mealtime and snack time, and stick to these whenever possible. However, flexibility is key. Don't fret over a change in schedule, but be aware of the adjustments to be made when, for example, a meal or snack is delayed, or an insulin injection is scheduled during a sports event.

- Involve your child in the routines, and acknowledge their feelings and concerns about diabetes. Encourage their mastery of the diabetes routines — choosing snacks and doing finger pricks and insulin injections.

- Try to control your own stresses, frustrations and anxieties surrounding diabetes. Children are sensitive to these displays and may either mirror your responses or try to hide things from you to avoid upsetting you. Seek support from the diabetes team, other parents of children with diabetes or a support group.

Adolescents

Adolescence is a time of rapid biological change, accompanied by increasing physical, cognitive and emotional maturity. It is a time of increasing peer conformity, experimentation, limit-testing and independence from family. Self-image changes with the emergence of sexuality, and the experience may be difficult and even frightening for some.

Even though it may seem that these young people should be more responsible, and more able to achieve "good" blood glucose control, adolescence is frequently the time when adequate blood glucose control is most difficult. Diabetes management requires a degree of responsibility and behavioral control that is uncharacteristic of many adolescents. The daily demands of the disease have an impact on the personal and public lives of teens, affecting important developmental areas including independence, body image, identity, sexuality, responsibility and self-esteem.

With or without diabetes, the progression of adolescent development varies greatly both across and within age groups, and within individuals. An important milestone is the acquisition of abstract reasoning, which allows the adolescent to understand fully the implications of diabetes and its management. There are, however, many compelling and conflicting factors — peer pressure, parties and other social events, part-time jobs and a busy life in general — that may interfere with the teen's ability to translate this new awareness into good self-care behaviors.

CASE HISTORY

Clear Expectations

Jackie is 14 and has had diabetes since the age of 7. She's proud of the fact that she manages her diabetes independently. She checks her blood glucose three or four times a day, and takes her insulin three times a day. Already she participates in decisions about insulin dose adjustment. Her A1c checks have been consistently in the 7s, indicating excellent blood glucose control. She's happy and involved in school and extracurricular activities.

At a recent clinic visit, the doctor discovered that, on one of the few occasions when Jackie's blood glucose checks were high, she recorded a lower result. When this was pointed out to Jackie, she became very tearful. With a little prompting, she told her diabetes nurse that she felt sad and upset because she was looking forward to a youth group trip to Ottawa, and her parents had agreed that she could go if she maintained "good" diabetes control; she believed that they wouldn't let her go if they saw the high blood glucose results. Jackie asked her nurse to help her explain the doctor's discovery and her feelings and concerns to her mother, who was in the waiting room.

As Jackie's mom listened to the explanation, tears welled up in her eyes. She put her arm around her daughter, saying, "Jackie, that's not what your father and I meant by 'good' control. We should have been clearer about what we expected." In fact, all her parents meant was that she should put in a strong effort. Everyone has occasional highs and lows, sometimes for no apparent reason, and Jackie's parents hadn't meant to suggest that they expected perfection. The misunderstanding created an opportunity for Jackie and her parents to clarify and renegotiate their goals.

Three Important Facts about Diabetes in Adolescents

1. **Insulin action:** The growth spurt of puberty is fueled by an increase in two hormones: insulin-like growth factor-1 (IGF-1) and growth hormone (GH). This leads to a decrease in insulin action in the liver, fat and muscle. In those without diabetes, the body responds by increasing insulin secretion, which helps lay down the protein, fat and carbohydrate stores, the building blocks of growth. In those with diabetes, increased insulin doses are required during this period. This may lead to increasing weight gain and more variability in blood glucose control with higher A1c levels. The increasing

levels of IGF-1 and GH may contribute significantly to the increased risk of onset and/or progression of diabetes-related complications during this critical time period of adolescence.

2. **"Behavior":** At the same time as there are biological reasons for changing insulin requirements and glucose control during puberty, so, too, are there behavioral changes as the youth progresses from late childhood toward adulthood. Typically, teens move from being family-oriented to being much more influenced by friends and trends. As an aside, the inability of parents to recognize this evolving independence is one cause of conflict.

Adolescence is also a time of experimentation and risk-taking behavior. Much of this relates to the teen's attempt to figure out their identity, and may manifest through their choice of clothes and music, or behaviors such as smoking, or use of alcohol and drugs. This is a time of delicate balance between parents and the evolving teen. Often, teens like to push back, at the same time needing the security of a sound home base. Parents need to recognize this and allow the teen increasing freedom while also providing a steadying hand.

Adolescence is clearly a time when the emerging teen goes through a significant period of personal development; parents and caregivers also must evolve in a way that supports the teen's personal growth. This is very difficult for some parents, and communication often breaks down.

3. **Outcomes:** A1c levels during the teen years tend to be about 1% to 1.5% higher on average than in younger children or adults. Research suggests that as many as 45% of teens with diabetes may exhibit troublesome behavior such as significant noncompliance with routines, school avoidance or dropout, depression and eating disorders.

Helping an Adolescent Deal with Diabetes

- Remain involved in your teen's diabetes care, at some level, right through adolescence. Diabetes management is a heavy burden to carry alone.

- Let go gradually. Make sure your teen is ready, willing and able to take on the aspects of diabetes management you are ready to give up.

Did You Know?
Teen-Speak

A teenager's language may consist of grunts and/or teen-speak when responding to questions. Teens respond to changes in cultural norms more rapidly than their parents, and this can make their language difficult to understand at times.

CASE HISTORY

The Keys to Success

There are a significant number of teens who navigate their way through adolescence without a hitch: excellent A1c levels, outstanding school performance and few if any conflicts at home. When asked to define their keys to success, the answer is always the same: "I dunno." Then they look at their doctor as if to say: Doesn't everyone do the same? Very recently, the mother of one of these teens said: "I know. He has a neurotic mother!" We can interpret her comment to mean that she is concerned and attentive, yet secure enough to have given her son plenty of room to grow and develop.

- Parents, teens and the diabetes team must all have the same expectations of the teen and of each other. Is everyone aiming for the same blood glucose target? Can everyone agree on the frequency of blood glucose monitoring? Can everyone agree about who chooses what foods at mealtime? Goals and expectations should be reviewed jointly, on a regular basis, to be sure they're still appropriate.

- All teens hate to be nagged, but most don't mind a little help. Parents can help get the monitoring equipment ready for a check, instead of simply saying, "It's that time again." Similarly, they can offer to keep the log, instead of complaining that they don't know what's going on because the numbers never get recorded in the book.

> **Pro Tip**
>
> Praise adolescents freely. There is no danger of giving them an inflated ego, and positive reinforcement will only yield more of the desired behavior.

- Be prepared to get re-involved as necessary. Even the most self-sufficient teen is going to need backup during particularly stressful periods, such as during a crisis in a relationship, an illness or a time of overwhelming competing priorities. This is not a step backward; it's just evidence of the family working together to ensure that the teen's health is maintained at all times.

- Teens should be encouraged to develop their own relationships with members of their diabetes team. Allow a teen private time with the doctor or educator at each clinic visit. It's natural for parents to want to stay informed, to have time to discuss issues and to be part of developing the plan for the next phase. However, teens should be able to expect confidentiality in certain aspects of their health care.

Why Teens Hate Checking Their Blood Glucose Levels

- It's inconvenient and time-consuming — to a teen, losing a few minutes of sleep or social time means a lot.

- Each check is a reminder that they have diabetes and are not the same as their peers.

- They feel accountable for each blood glucose result — parents frequently demand explanations for high or low readings.

- The results may make them feel guilty — they may know why they're high but be unwilling to do anything about it. It feels better not to check.

- They don't understand the purpose of checking — they don't know how to use the results.

- They feel discouraged by the results, which don't reflect their efforts to manage their diabetes.

It's worthwhile having a discussion with your teen in an attempt to discover what the issues are in their particular case.

Respecting Privacy and Confidentiality

Time alone with their health care professionals enables teens to ask questions they may feel uncomfortable asking with their parents in the room.

As adolescents mature, they need to have some time alone with their health care professionals. This should be offered and respected by the parents. It enables the teens to ask questions they may feel uncomfortable asking with their parents in the room. This forms the basis of the teen developing autonomy, defined in this case as "self-directing freedom and especially moral independence."

Being alone with the teen also affords the opportunity for team members to broach subjects that teens need to start thinking about. It is important that the teens understand, however, that their diabetes team members will need to share information if action or inaction could lead to a situation that may be dangerous for the teen. Confidentiality can only be breached when there is severe hypoglycemia that might occur while driving or if there is a history of abuse or neglect.

Special Considerations in the Teenage Years

Smoking, drug and alcohol abuse, eating disorders and unprotected sex that leads to pregnancy are recognized hazards.

Did You Know?
Sometimes Less Is More

For some teens, there are occasions when "less is more." For example, if repeated attempts at improving a teen's glucose levels have failed, it may be time to step back and simplify the treatment routine rather than offering increasingly complex solutions (more frequent injections, complex dose adjustment routines, et cetera) that are being ignored. Ask the teen what they think they could accomplish during the next interval between clinic visits. *Listen carefully* to their answer, and take baby steps that can be easily incorporated into a simplified routine.

However, teens with diabetes must be fully aware of the problems associated with these behaviors and the additional risks to their health. The use of alcohol, for example, increases the risk of severe hypoglycemia, and smoking greatly increases the chance of early stroke, heart attack and other diabetes-related complications. It is impossible to make wise choices without accurate information.

It is also critical for parents to understand that diabetes routines may become a target for risk-taking behavior. Teens may skip meals or blood glucose checks. Some may even skip their insulin. If such behavior seriously compromises diabetes control, resulting in poor school attendance, hospitalization (due to diabetic ketoacidosis) or poor growth or weight loss, parents will need to resume giving the injections and supervising blood glucose checks, regardless of the teen's age, until there is evidence that it's safe to allow the teen to manage independently once again.

Smoking

Everyone knows the horrifying consequences of smoking: chronic lung disease and lung cancer; heart disease and other vascular problems; poor exercise performance; and much more.

Many teens try cigarettes. Unfortunately, some become regular users. Given that diabetes and smoking both target the small blood vessels of the body, the results are predictable: earlier and more severe diabetes-related complications in those who choose to smoke compared to those who do not. This is an issue that needs anticipatory guidance starting before puberty, with more information and help provided along the way. Better not to start smoking than to try to stop later.

Did You Know?
Online Resources

For the American Diabetes Association's position on smoking and diabetes, visit www.diabetes.org/ are-you-at-risk/ lower-your-risk/ smoking.html. For Diabetes Canada recommendations, see www.diabetes. ca/diabetes-and- you/healthy- living-resources/ heart-health/ smoking-diabetes.

Peer influences may be stronger than those of the parents both in starting and stopping smoking. Teens who have already started smoking may benefit from a smoking cessation program offered at school or perhaps at an adolescent medicine clinic or public health unit.

Alcohol

Alcohol interferes with the liver's ability to produce glucose from its stores and release it into the blood.

There are a few truths about alcohol and diabetes. First, alcohol use is illegal below 18 to 21 years of age in most places. Nonetheless, many teens experiment with alcohol despite the legalities. Alcohol is available in many places and easy to obtain in our societies. Second, alcohol interferes with the liver's ability to produce glucose from its stores and release it into the blood. This creates a serious risk of low blood glucose, or hypoglycemia. The effects of alcohol and low glucose may be similar, and smelling alcohol on the breath will likely mean overlooking the possibility of hypoglycemia and blaming the behavior on excessive alcohol use. Furthermore, under the influence of alcohol, a teen may miss the early warning symptoms of hypoglycemia and progress quickly to a severe episode.

Advice for Teens Planning to Drink

- Drink in moderation and be sure at least one of the group does not drink and is able to serve as a "designated driver" or otherwise offer help.

- Always be sure to eat something substantial when drinking.

- Check blood glucose levels before going to bed and do not sleep in too late the following morning.

   In other words, be sensible, be moderate and do not drink and drive!

Marijuana and Other Drugs

Different mood-enhancing drugs can have very different effects on diabetes control. Since all of these drugs are mind-altering, it is very important to have people around who are not using the drug in order to help if needed. Best advice: say no to drugs!

Marijuana impairs the judgment required to recognize and acknowledge the signs of low blood glucose. Marijuana use also triggers food cravings and hunger — the "munchies" — leading to overeating, which can, in turn, cause high blood glucose.

The direct effect of other street drugs on blood glucose level is not well known. They may do other damage and may also contribute to impaired judgment and risk-taking behaviors such as unprotected intercourse.

Sex and Contraception

Sexually active teens require contraception to prevent unplanned pregnancies. Generally speaking, the same options are available to women with diabetes as to those without. Even women who take an oral contraceptive should require their partner to use a condom in order to reduce the risk of sexually transmitted infections.

All sexually active teens should consider intercourse as an extra activity that uses up energy, requiring a carbohydrate snack afterward.

Teens with diabetes should be provided with information about sexuality, contraception and pregnancy well in advance of needing it. These discussions should take place with members of the diabetes team and should be confidential.

Eating Disorders

Eating disorders are common among teenage and young adult women and are much less common among males in the same age group. Researchers believe they stem from an obsession about gaining control in a life they perceive to be out of control. There are many possible causes of this obsession, depending on the individual's experience. People with anorexia nervosa try to regain control by denying themselves food; people with bulimia nervosa try to regain control by excessive overeating (binging), and then purging by self-induced vomiting or with the aid of laxatives. These definitions aren't cut-and-dried — people with one disorder sometimes exhibit characteristics of the other. In the long term, anorexia can lead to severe weight loss and can be fatal. The constant binging and purging of bulimia can result in severe stomach ulcers and can also be fatal.

In teenage and young adult women with type 1 diabetes, disturbances in eating attitudes and behavior are common and persistent. Full-blown eating disorders occur in as many as 10% of teenage girls with diabetes, but even milder disturbances can wreak havoc with blood glucose control.

Some diabetes-related factors may increase the likelihood of an eating disturbance. At the time of diagnosis, there is often weight loss. With insulin therapy, this weight is quickly regained. In the vulnerable girl, this may trigger dissatisfaction with her body and the desire to be thinner again. Also, meal planning is an integral part of diabetes treatment.

Such planning implies a degree of dietary restraint, another trigger to disordered eating. Finally, some girls discover that by skipping or reducing their insulin dose, they can lose glucose in their urine and keep themselves underweight. Although this may be an effective way to control weight, it invariably leads to poor diabetes control and, in the long run, earlier onset of diabetes-related complications.

Full-blown eating disorders occur in as many as 10% of teenage girls with diabetes, but even milder disturbances can wreak havoc with blood glucose control.

Warnings Signs of an Eating Disorder

Eating disorders in people with type 1 diabetes can lead to wild, unexplained fluctuations in blood glucose levels, often outside the safe range. Frequent low glucose reactions (insulin reactions) or high glucose reactions (excessive thirst and urination, perhaps leading to urinary ketones) may be a sign that an eating disorder is complicating diabetes management. Eating disorders can also be marked by:

- A preoccupation with food and weight, beyond what is required in diabetes management
- A stated desire to lose weight beyond what seems appropriate
- Requests for dietary change with low-calorie, low-fat, vegetarian or other diets to lose weight
- Binge-eating episodes
- Insulin manipulation

What You Can Do to Help

If your child has an eating disorder, there are several things you can do to help.

- Express your concern for their health while respecting the need for privacy. Eating disorders are usually a symptom of a greater psychological problem, and the fact that you are there to help will be appreciated.
- Examine your own attitudes around food and weight. Are you furthering the idea that "thin is in"?
- Talk about more flexible meal plans with your diabetes dietitian. Perhaps the current meal plan is too restrictive, reinforcing the idea that your child is different and deprived.
- Avoid commenting on weight, either positively or negatively, as it only serves to emphasize the importance of appearance.
- Express your concern to your diabetes health care team and get support for your child.

Driving

Driving a car requires accurate judgment and a keen sense of responsibility. Young people with diabetes have an additional responsibility to ensure that their blood glucose is in the right range before they get behind the wheel of a car. Low blood glucose can impair judgment, increasing the risk of an accident. Parents should be certain that teens show responsible self-management before permitting them to apply for a driver's license or lending them the family vehicle.

Getting a regular driver's license is not generally a problem, as long as blood glucose control is reasonable and there have been no severe episodes of hypoglycemia in the previous year. People living with diabetes are eligible for a commercial driver's license. (See Further Resources, "Driving and Diabetes," for more information.)

Pro Tip

Avoid power struggles around food. Forcing someone with an eating disorder to eat will probably make things worse.

Diabetes and Driving

Low blood glucose can affect one's judgment and level of consciousness while driving.

All drivers with diabetes:

- Should measure their blood glucose level immediately before and at least every four hours during long drives, and more often if they have hypoglycemia (low blood glucose) unawareness

- Should always carry a meter and supplies of fast-acting carbohydrate within easy reach in the car

- Should stop and treat as soon as they sense hypoglycemia or have difficulty driving

Blood glucose level before driving:

- If blood glucose is below 72 mg/dL (4 mmol/L), treat with 15 grams of carbohydrate, wait 15 minutes and make sure blood glucose is above 90 mg/dL (5 mmol/L) before driving.

- If blood glucose is 72 to 90 mg/dL (4 to 5 mmol/L), treat with 15 grams of carbohydrate to prevent it from going lower.

- Blood glucose should be above 90 mg/dL (5 mmol/L) before you drive.

Following these recommendations and taking steps to avoid severe hypoglycemia during the day are necessary in order to maintain a driver's license.

Near the time for applying for a driver's permit, we recommend that a member of the diabetes team review the team's recommendations regarding driving, then have the teen sign the form to signify that they have understood these instructions.

Source: Recommendations from the American Diabetes Association and Diabetes Canada

Employment

There are countless examples of people with diabetes who have excelled in a broad range of careers — doctors, lawyers, nurses, politicians, professional athletes, psychologists, accountants, researchers, teachers and engineers, to mention a few. In general, parents and educators find that young people can be coached and counseled to pursue the career that interests them or for which they have an aptitude. However, it is also important to be aware of current limitations. Two questions are often asked of the diabetes team: "Are there jobs that are not available to people with diabetes?" and "Do some employers discriminate against people with diabetes?" The answer to both questions is *yes*.

A number of organizations once had blanket rules preventing employment of people with diabetes. Such employment includes jobs that require operation of a commercial vehicle, such as a truck or an aircraft, and jobs in some military or police departments. These rules were based on the risk of hypoglycemia while on the job. When applying for a particular educational or employment opportunity, teens with diabetes should inquire as to their employability in these areas. However, blanket rules excluding people with diabetes from certain jobs or from obtaining a commercial vehicle license have been replaced by screening questionnaires. (See Further Resources, "Driving and Diabetes," for more information.)

Employer discrimination has been documented over many years. There is often a misconception that people with diabetes will attend their jobs less frequently and perform less effectively than their peers. Young job seekers with diabetes should stress their personal qualifications, abilities and ambitions to potential employers. They should not withhold information about their diabetes, but rather stress the fact that they can perform as well as others. If they believe they are being treated unfairly, they should seek advice through their advocacy group, such as the American Diabetes Association or Diabetes Canada.

> Young job seekers with diabetes should stress their personal qualifications, abilities and ambitions to potential employers.

Helpful Hints for All Ages

- Get everyone in the family involved. Diabetes care is a partnership between the child or teen and the entire family. In two-parent families, mothers often shoulder a major share of the responsibility, but fathers need to take part as well. Talk about your feelings in an open manner.

On the other hand, try not to let diabetes become the focus of every family meal or discussion. Also, recruit the support of others — grandparents, camp counselors, teachers and coaches. The more they know about your child, the more comfortable you'll feel when they're in charge.

- Set realistic blood glucose targets. Expecting every blood glucose to be, say, 145 mg/dL (8 mmol/L) is unrealistic. In fact, it's impossible! Good diabetes control means balancing all aspects of your life and lifestyle, not just focusing on blood glucose results.

- Make good use of your diabetes team. Don't be afraid to ask questions — and ask more questions if the answers don't seem to fit. (See chapter 11 for more about getting the most out of your diabetes team.)

- Take credit for trying, and don't feel bad about mistakes — they're bound to happen. Diabetes is a complex and often frustrating condition. Doing the same thing two days in a row does not always lead to the same results.

- Experiment a little and see what works for you and your child. What you learn in your diabetes education and clinic sessions provides you with an excellent foundation. You've become an expert in your own child's diabetes. But you haven't been given every answer to every question. Also, some things work better for some people. Use your knowledge to experiment a little. For example, taking less insulin before a sports game may work better in a particular situation than eating a large amount of extra food.

- Be realistic in your expectations of what responsibility your child will take for the diabetes. Don't expect too much too soon. On the other hand, try not to be overbearing and overprotective.

- Be sure to praise good performance. It's very easy to focus on the negatives. "You're late for your blood glucose check!" "Did you take your insulin yet?" It's also easy to overlook the positives. Rather, praise every little advance, and look for opportunities for ongoing education when things are a little offtrack.

Q & A

Q. It takes half an hour of bargaining to get my 3-year-old to cooperate during injection time. How can I make this go more smoothly?

A. It's not unusual for children of all ages to go through periods when they cry, squirm and use all kinds of delaying tactics to avoid insulin injections and finger pricks. Sometimes they are angry about being held still or having their play interrupted. Remember how hard it is just to wipe a toddler's nose! They may also be reacting to the fear and anxiety they sense in you. Here are some helpful hints for making injection time go more smoothly:

- Try to take a matter-of-fact approach to the insulin injections and finger pricks.
- Be quick, calm and reassuring when you carry out these routines.
- Reduce your child's anxious time by getting the dose and/or equipment ready before you involve the child.
  - If possible, go to where the child is playing to cause less disruption.
  - Gently hold or restrain your child if they struggle.
  - Get the needle or finger prick over with quickly. Delaying it only prolongs the agony for everyone.
  - Give your child a big hug and kiss after you give the needle, even if they didn't cooperate.
  - Praise your child for any sign of cooperation.

Pro Tip

Your child's crying, protests and other delaying tactics are normal. Remember that, each time you give insulin or do a finger prick, you are helping your child stay healthy.

Q. Can diabetes complicate menstruation?

A. No, but the hormonal increase prior to or during menstruation can cause blood glucose levels to rise. Some women require more insulin just before or during their periods. This is checked by observing the blood glucose pattern during the menstrual cycle.

Q. Can my teen sleep in on weekends?

A. Although your diabetes team stresses consistency in the timing of meals and snacks, with a little extra effort and caution, your teen can make the adjustments needed to sleep in safely. For example, if they are going to bed at midnight on Saturday night and want to sleep in until 10 a.m. Sunday, try this: instead of taking evening NPH insulin at 10 p.m., take it at midnight, together with a blood glucose check and a little extra snack. This will help decrease the risk of low blood glucose levels during those extra sleep hours.

If your teen is on an MDI insulin routine or an insulin pump, sleeping in is much easier. He should stay on his overnight basal rate and take a bolus with his first meal. If your teen isn't using either one of these treatment routines but needs more flexibility, switching to these regimens should be considered.

Q. I have a hard time getting my teen to do a blood glucose check. I know from attending a parents' group meeting that other parents have the same problem. To avoid this conflict, can we decrease the number of checks he needs to do every day?

A. It is often said about adolescence that it is just a phase that will pass, and that, in those with type 1 diabetes, things will get better as they move into young adulthood. This is an incorrect approach for many reasons: first, teens with deteriorating metabolic control put themselves at risk of diabetic ketoacidosis and exposure to significant persistent hyperglycemia, predisposing them to an earlier than expected onset of complications. Second, the risk to complication development is contributed to by the duration and severity of the hyperglycemia during the early pubertal years, a risk that might not be countered by improving control as adulthood is reached. Finally, poor metabolic control during adolescence is a serious risk factor for ongoing poor control into adulthood.

There is no surefire way of ensuring that your teen does their blood glucose testing on a regular basis. But taking a nonjudgmental approach, avoiding shame and blame, praising even small achievements and offering to assist them where possible may help in the long run.

> Poor metabolic control during adolescence is a serious risk factor for ongoing poor control into adulthood.

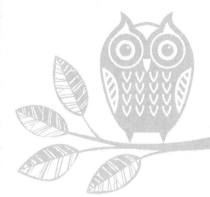

Chapter 10

Diabetes Outside the Home

Learning how to incorporate diabetes care into settings outside of the home will help greatly to empower children and teens.

As children and teens grow and develop, they spend more and more time outside their homes, in increasingly less closely supervised situations. Since there is no break in the need for diabetes care, the involvement of others is necessary for children to be safe and have successful management while they are busy enjoying other aspects of their life, such as school, extracurricular activities and time with family and friends. This chapter aims to help you prepare others and eventually your child themselves to "fit" diabetes care into important everyday social settings.

Key Messages

- Specific details of diabetes management need to be communicated to other caregivers, depending on their level of involvement.

- Children can start to take on more responsibility for their diabetes care both at home and outside the home, depending on their age, maturity level and demonstrated ability to follow through with these routines.

- With careful planning, learning how to incorporate diabetes care into settings outside of the home will help greatly to empower children and teens, as well as other caregivers.

In the Classroom

The demands of diabetes management cannot help but have an impact on school life. School personnel must be aware of the student with diabetes and, depending on their level of involvement, understand specific care needs and how they can ensure the student's safety. This applies not only in the classroom but also in the playground, on school trips and in sports activities. By understanding the relevant aspects of diabetes management, the teacher can also ensure the student's healthy adjustment to the classroom setting and peer interactions.

A knowledgeable and supportive teacher will help calm parental anxiety and will prevent minor crises from getting out of control. But a poorly informed or misinformed teacher — one who perhaps has great anxiety about having a student with diabetes in the classroom — can add to the adjustment and management difficulties encountered by the child or teen and the family.

Step 1: Establish and Maintain Good Communication with the School

When parents or alternate caregivers first inform the school about their child's or teen's diabetes diagnosis, they will often encounter variable levels of knowledge and comfort in how to best support their child within this setting. This is understandable, since it is unrealistic to expect the majority of teachers to be well informed about every potential health condition. However, when a student with a health condition does come under their care at school, teachers and school personnel should gain the necessary know-how to be able to provide reliable and capable support. What this looks like will depend on the student's age, stage of development and diabetes care routines.

Regardless of your child's age, it is necessary to arrange a meeting with their teachers and other school personnel as soon after diagnosis as possible to discuss their new diabetes management needs. This meeting will need to occur again at the beginning of each school year, due to changes in treatment plans (for example, if a child moves from an injection regimen to an insulin pump) and maturity level, which could affect how involved and responsible the child or teen is in their diabetes routines. At these times, provide teachers with the appropriate information about your child's diabetes care, and make sure to update them if this plan changes during the school year.

Your diabetes team should provide you with current resources about managing diabetes at school. The American Diabetes Association has a *Safe At School* resource (www.diabetes.org/living-with-diabetes/parents-and-kids/diabetes-care-at-school). In Canada, www.diabetesatschool.ca is an excellent online resource with many written information sheets and online videos.

Did You Know?
Diabetes Care Mandates

Countries differ in the laws regarding diabetes care at school: some mandate that school personnel administer insulin and/or have funding to support school nurses, while others do not. This is something to discuss with your diabetes team while planning for your child's diabetes care at school.

Step 2: Clarify What the School Needs to Know

> One of the most important things for teachers to know about diabetes is how to recognize hypoglycemia and prevent a mild low blood glucose from turning into a more severe one.

Teachers and other school personnel are not health care professionals, but since children are with them for the majority of the day on weekdays, they do have a significant role to play in supporting students and ensuring their safety. One of the most important things for teachers to know about diabetes is how to recognize hypoglycemia and prevent a mild low blood glucose from turning into a more severe one. In order to recognize hypoglycemia, the school needs to know the child's specific low blood glucose symptoms or what the potential symptoms could be (in the case of a child who has just recently been diagnosed with diabetes). As well, the teacher and/or principal should ensure that other school personnel who also come into contact with your child are aware of these symptoms, especially so they won't be mistaken for "not paying attention" or "acting out."

It is also vital that staff know what to do if your child feels or acts like they are experiencing a low blood glucose. This includes first verifying these symptoms with an actual blood glucose check — it's important to ensure everyone knows where the meter is kept and that the necessary treatment is available at school. Ideally, these supplies are accessible in the child's classroom. In some circumstances, they can be kept in the office; if this is the case, a plan should be in place for a "buddy" to accompany your child to this spot if they are experiencing hypoglycemia.

School staff should also become familiar with the signs of high blood glucose, or hyperglycemia, and notify parents if the child has to leave the classroom to go to the bathroom more frequently than usual. When to contact parents regarding high blood glucose should be outlined in the child's specific diabetes plan, and details will often vary depending on the child's insulin regimen and age. Parents should definitely be contacted right away if their child is unwell with a high blood glucose that includes symptoms such as nausea, abdominal pain and/or vomiting. If the child vomits, the parents or another designated responsible adult should be notified. If that person is unavailable, a plan for what school personnel should do next should be outlined in your child's individual care plan (for example, contact diabetes team, take to closest emergency room).

Hypoglycemia in Young Students

Teachers of younger children need to be especially observant during gym/recess periods and remind the child with diabetes to take a snack. They should ensure that children have time to eat their lunch and snacks as well, since missing food at these times will likely lead to preventable hypoglycemia. If a teacher is not present when a younger child is eating their lunch, staff that supervise during this time also need to be involved in supporting the younger child to eat their lunch and in communicating if there were any issues.

Teachers should also understand that meal plans are an important element of diabetes care and that without advance notice it can be hard for children with diabetes to participate in surprise pizza parties or snacks. Teachers should inform parents of any such events so the child's meal plan and insulin dose can be adjusted accordingly. They should also be aware of the need for between-meal snacks.

Step 3: Determine the Exact Involvement of the School

In general, the involvement of teachers in providing direct diabetes care can be quite variable and requires a discussion between parents and school personnel. From this conversation, an agreement needs to be outlined in the child's individual care plan. At the very least, school personnel should understand enough about the diabetes care routines so that they can supply any necessary supervision or, alternatively, allow the child privacy to do injections and blood glucose testing.

As well, the school should have a plan of action outlined in the student's individual care plan in case the child has severe hypoglycemic symptoms (being unresponsive or unconscious, having a seizure, refusing juice or sugar by mouth) while at school. In general, the school should be able to respond to severe hypoglycemia symptoms by:

1. Placing the student in the recovery position.

2. Calling emergency services (911).

3. Giving glucagon only if there is a signed consent and mutual agreement between the school and parents. Staff who are identified as able to give this medication need to be trained. This information should be clearly outlined in the student's individual care plan.

HOW TO: Help the School Be Prepared to Identify and Treat Hypoglycemia

1. Provide school staff with a written resource of the signs and symptoms of hypoglycemia.

2. Inform school staff of your child's specific low blood glucose symptoms.

3. Have low blood glucose treatments stocked at school and make sure there is a designated spot where these are kept. Restock throughout the year as necessary.

4. Have equipment available to check blood glucose at school (glucose monitor, test strips, lancets) and ensure school staff and your child are aware of the location of these supplies.

5. Create a means for communicating if a low blood glucose occurred at school.

Field Trips

Children with diabetes should be encouraged to participate in as many school activities as they choose and should not be excluded from school trips. However, planning ahead is essential. If your child or teen is participating in physical activities beyond those they do on a daily basis, extra food should be packed in their knapsack or lunch box. Include a mix of fast-acting carbohydrate snacks, such as juice boxes and dried fruit, to prevent low glucose episodes, and carbohydrate snacks such as crackers and granola bars.

Careful preparation for overnight trips or special events will help prevent problems. If the event — for example, a field trip to the zoo — overlaps an insulin injection or blood test time, ensure that one of the teachers or chaperoning parents takes responsibility for either performing or supervising the task. Children and accompanying adults should always have supplies to treat low blood glucose, such as juice, glucose tablets or even a glucagon kit for overnight or longer trips. Children should know how to recognize symptoms of low blood glucose before they are permitted to go on overnight field trips. Before that, consider volunteering as a chaperone yourself.

> Children and accompanying adults should always have supplies to treat low blood glucose, such as juice, glucose tablets or even a glucagon kit for overnight or longer trips.

WHAT TO: Pack on a Field Trip

On field trips of any type, in addition to an informed adult companion, the child with diabetes must have:

- A source of fast-acting concentrated carbohydrate to treat hypoglycemia (for example, juice boxes, glucose tablets, hard candy)

- Visible identification that indicates that they have diabetes, such as a medical-alert bracelet

- Insulin, syringes/pens (or pump supplies) and blood testing equipment, if the trip overlaps a testing or injection time

- The phone number of a parent or an informed responsible adult

Summer Camp

For many school-age children and teens, summertime means not only a holiday from school, but also the opportunity to play and spend time with friends at either day camps or sleepover camps. For children with diabetes, the situation is no different, and with proper planning, they, too, can enjoy a fun-filled, healthy and safe camp experience.

Day Camps

The preparation for day camps is similar to the preparation for a family day out or a day trip at school. Make sure your child has all meals and snacks prepared and packed. For most children, minor adjustments in timing allow all insulin injections to be given at home as usual (the exception is children who are on a lunchtime injection and are able to administer it themselves). Similarly, at least three daily blood glucose tests can be performed at home, and blood glucose levels can be monitored by a parent. Children should do a prelunch glucose check at camp.

Ask camp staff about the level of activity in which your child will participate. Inform them that your child has diabetes and emphasize the importance of the timing of food intake. The signs and symptoms of hypoglycemia should be explained, and a source of rapid-acting glucose should be supplied to a counselor to treat a low blood glucose episode. Furthermore, the camp staff must, like teachers, be told what to do in the event of a severe hypoglycemic episode.

Overnight Camps

What about overnight camps? Are they safe for children with diabetes? Absolutely. However, to provide a happy and safe camping experience and to ensure that the principles of daily diabetes care are followed, the American Diabetes Association, Diabetes Canada and several other organizations have set up camps especially for children and teens with diabetes. Whenever possible, children and teens with diabetes should have the chance to attend such camps. They are usually staffed by doctors and nurses experienced in the care of children with diabetes. In addition, an experienced dietitian is there to assist the children in meal planning. The programming staff is accustomed to working with campers with diabetes and develops programs to match the timing of daily diabetes routines. With such a support system, the children can enjoy the full range of camp experiences — including swimming, boating, tripping, crafts and drama — without the burden of managing their diabetes care alone.

These camps also give children the opportunity to spend several days or weeks with other campers who have diabetes. Having spent most of the school year with children who do not have diabetes, many campers are excited to be with other kids like them. Everybody is doing blood checks, testing urine, taking insulin injections, monitoring diet and watching for low blood glucose episodes. Some children learn to give their own injections for the first time under the direction of the camp nurse and with the encouragement of their summer friends. For others, especially those from smaller communities, this may be their first experience of not being the only child with diabetes.

Some children and teens prefer to go to camps not specifically aimed at those with diabetes. If the child or teen has sufficient knowledge, sense of responsibility and willingness to monitor the condition, this, too, can be accommodated by proper planning.

Involving Babysitters, Family, Friends and Other Caregivers

Expanding your diabetes "circle of friends" is important in order to provide you with added support and also to help your child know that other trusted people can also help them take care of their diabetes. It may take you a little while after your child is diagnosed to let others be involved; however, during this time, you can think about what your family and close friends can do to support you while you get used to helping your child with their daily diabetes tasks. This could include helping out with your other children, doing an errand for you or just lending an ear if you're feeling overwhelmed or worried.

On an ongoing basis, try to involve others when it's time to give an injection. It's also important to prepare others for unpredictable events and offer instructions on what to do in these particular situations, such as recognizing and treating a low blood glucose. Then, when both you and your child are ready to be apart, you will have others who are prepared to be involved and can step in without having to start at the beginning in learning about your child's specific diabetes care.

Important Details to Share with Others Caring for Your Child

- The timing of meals and snacks (depending on your child's age and involvement, you may need to provide specific details on what to prepare at these times)

- The low blood glucose symptoms your child typically experiences; what constitutes a low blood glucose reading on the meter; and the specific treatment and follow-up plan once hypoglycemia has been identified

- The timing of blood glucose monitoring, insulin injection times and dose amounts (level of involvement will vary depending on child's age and ability)

- Contact information and instructions on when to be in touch immediately

Remember that most children attending camp are more active than usual and have less access to food between meals. As a result, they may require a lower or different insulin dose to avoid hypoglycemic episodes. More frequent blood glucose monitoring will be needed to determine the actual insulin requirement. Whenever possible, choose a camp with a full-time physician and nurse on site who can help deal with diabetes routines and any illness that may occur.

Planning for Physical Activity

Diabetes aside, physical activity is something that all children should be involved in on a daily basis, not only for the positive short- and long-term health outcomes, but also for an overall feeling of both social and mental well-being. Whether it involves going for a bike ride with friends, a weekly recreational sport or a high-level competitive league, children with diabetes should not be limited in what activities they choose to try and possibly what sport they may end up excelling at.

As discussed in chapter 3, incorporating exercise into the routine of a child who has diabetes does require a carefully thought-out plan and often detailed monitoring, due to the varying effects of physical activity on blood glucose levels. There is likely no such thing as a "perfect formula"; however, each family eventually develops an understanding of how they are able to best manage their own child's blood glucose levels during their particular activity. As well, with more recent advances in **continuous glucose monitoring systems** (CGMS) and experience in using insulin pump therapy among athletes with diabetes, there are now readily available tools and information that you can use to better understand the effects of activity in your own child (see Further Resources, "Exercise and Diabetes," for more specific references).

Effects of Exercise on Blood Glucose Levels

Before outlining some strategies to try when your child begins to exercise after being diagnosed with diabetes, or joins a new sport at a later time, it's helpful to remember how the body regulates blood glucose levels during exercise in people without and with type 1 diabetes.

Without Type 1 Diabetes

When exercise starts, the glucose stored within the muscles is used to provide the initial burst of energy required. Once this is used up, more glucose goes into the cells from the bloodstream.

In order to do this, the body essentially switches off insulin secretion in order to allow the liver to deliver the needed glucose into the bloodstream from its stores. In addition, the counter-regulatory hormones, especially glucagon and adrenaline, are secreted in order to further increase the availability of glucose. The result is that, in those without diabetes, blood glucose levels remain stable throughout even prolonged exercise.

With Type 1 Diabetes

Exercise increases the amount of glucose your muscles use for energy. However, the pancreas is unable to produce insulin and can't lower injected insulin during exercise. In addition, counter-regulatory hormones may be higher, or even lower, which makes the normal regulation of glucose more difficult. As a result, blood glucose levels during activity often may decrease too much because of the presence of the injected or infused insulin, or increase too much due to the stress of the exercise.

There are many factors that impact the effects of exercise. All are important to consider when setting up a plan to manage your child's blood glucose during these times:

- **Duration of exercise:** Most exercise that lasts 30 minutes or more will need a plan to prevent a decrease in blood glucose levels.
- **Type of exercise:** Anaerobic activity (see "Terminology," at right) generally *increases* blood glucose levels for 30 to 60 minutes, due to the release of hormones, and is followed by lower blood glucose many hours later. Aerobic activity often lowers the blood glucose *during* the activity and for up to 7 to 11 hours following.
- **Type and timing of insulin injections:** If the action of the insulin is "peaking" during activity, there is more risk of hypoglycemia during this time.
- **Injection site:** If a site such as an arm or leg has been injected with insulin and is then exercised vigorously, the increased blood flow to this particular spot will result in faster absorption and insulin effect.

Adjusting Food and Insulin during Activity

Because exercise both typically lowers blood glucose and increases the speed of insulin absorption, it's a good idea to match it, whenever possible, with extra food and/or decreased insulin amounts. The aim of this book is to help families begin to plan for extra activity — not to lay out a detailed plan of

Monitor blood glucose levels before and after the activity; these levels will provide important information for future activities.

Terminology

Exercise can be either anaerobic or aerobic. Anaerobic activities feature brief, intense bursts of physical activity — for example, weight-lifting or sprinting. Aerobic activities are continuous exercises that increase the heart and breathing rate, but in a way that can be sustained for the exercise session — for example, running, swimming or walking.

how to adequately fuel a high-performance athlete with type 1 diabetes, which is much more complex and individualized (see Further Resources, "Exercise and Diabetes," for more direction on this type of planning). This being said, regardless of the type and level of your child's activity, in time you will become more familiar with how your child responds and what plan best works.

(see Further Resources, "Exercise and Diabetes," for more direction on this type of planning).

- In general, provide extra food for extra exercise. Children need about 10 to 15 grams of carbohydrate (such as a 4-ounce/125 mL juice box, or half a sandwich) for every 30 minutes of activity outside the usual. Monitor blood glucose levels before and after the activity; these levels will provide important information for future activities. For example, if the glucose level is very high after an activity, less (or no) extra food may be needed. If the glucose level is low, even more carbohydrate and/or a decrease in an insulin dose could be required.

- Examine your child's normal insulin routine to see if the "peak" action occurs during activity. Generally, in order to prevent hypoglycemia, a decrease in fast-acting insulin is necessary before activity that lasts 30 minutes or more. Reductions in long-acting insulin may be necessary, particularly if activity occurs later in the evening, before bed.

Tips for Preventing Hypoglycemia around Exercise

- Always make sure children have enough rapid-acting glucose with them (such as glucose tablets, Fruit Roll-Ups, juice boxes or granola bars), especially if the activity goes on a long time or is off the beaten track. This includes having these treatment options "on the bench" at games and making sure your child and coach know where these treatment sources are.

- If your child starts to experience low blood glucose symptoms, make sure they know to stop the activity immediately, check their blood glucose and treat. Let them know that they shouldn't restart the activity until they've eaten extra food and they feel better.

- Children doing activities after supper should have a larger evening snack. Doing a midnight or middle-of-the-night (2 to 4 a.m.) check will help detect late-night lows. In general, monitoring blood glucose long after a new exercise has started is important, since lows can occur up to 12 hours later.

CASE HISTORY

Preparing for Extra Activity

Ten-year-old Zoie's gymnastics class is normally on Saturday afternoon. She is currently on an MDI regimen. With her usual extra activity, Zoie often has more carbohydrate (15 grams extra) prior to the class, in addition to the minimal amount she usually has for her afternoon snack, which keeps her blood glucose levels in the 145 to 220 mg/L (8 to 12 mmol/L) range. However, this weekend she is involved in a competition that will begin midmorning and finish just before dinner. In preparation for this extra activity, Zoie's parents consider her current routine, which involves taking fast-acting insulin three times daily before meals and long-acting basal insulin before bedtime. Since this competition will likely mean that Zoie will be active during the time when both her morning and lunchtime fast-acting insulin (Humalog) will be working, Zoie's family plans the following:

1. *Take blood glucose meter to the competition so that extra checks can be done midmorning and midafternoon.*
2. *Pack low blood glucose treatment options that Zoie can keep in her gym bag and access easily as needed.*
3. *Decrease Zoie's fast-acting insulin doses by 20% at breakfast and lunchtime, since her blood glucose readings usually decrease with activity and she requires extra carbohydrate with her class.*
4. *Watch her blood glucose readings at dinner and bedtime and if they are in target, give a larger snack before bed that includes a protein option.*
5. *Check Zoie's blood glucose overnight due to the extra activity during the day and the potential for it to continue to affect Zoie's blood glucose levels.*

Keeping Track to Reevaluate the Plan

Whatever your child's involvement in activity, it is important to keep track of a few important things, which include:

- The timing of the activity
- The type of activity
- The carbohydrate eaten before, during and after the activity
- The blood glucose levels before, during and after the activity

At first, you will likely set up a plan with your diabetes team. Following that, your ongoing record-keeping will help you to better set up an individualized plan specific to your child. As well, depending on your child's level of exercise, you may decide to use CGMS technology or consider insulin pump therapy as a better means to adjust insulin doses more accurately with fluctuations in blood glucose levels.

Traveling with Diabetes

Diabetes should not limit your family's travels or be a barrier for the future experiences you anticipated for your child. Although it can take a while before you feel comfortable traveling, most families feel empowered following a first successful travel experience.

Unfortunately, you can't take a vacation from diabetes, and careful planning is essential to make sure traveling is safe and enjoyable. Here are some quick tips to help you prepare:

- Take enough insulin and other supplies to last for the entire trip, and some to spare. Keep the extra insulin in a separate location from the main supply in case one of your bags is lost or stolen. Bring an insulated bag to keep your insulin cool (especially your extra supplies).

- Be prepared for emergencies. Take a glucagon kit and ketone strips with you so you will have what you need if an illness or severe low blood glucose occurs. Give strong consideration to purchasing travel insurance, in case of accident or illness.

- Other countries may not recognize your prescriptions for medications; therefore, ensure you know how to obtain insulin and diabetes supplies in the country you are traveling to in the event that your insulin or supplies become lost or damaged. Some countries may require your child to be assessed by a local physician before they issue a prescription. Having proper travel insurance can help prevent financial burden.

- Take a letter (from a member of your diabetes team) explaining the need to carry sharps, juice boxes, et cetera, through airport security.

- If you're boarding a plane, make sure all your supplies are in your carry-on baggage. Even consider splitting the supplies between more than one piece of carry-on luggage.

- Wherever you go, always carry some food, together with a good supply of fast-acting glucose to treat hypoglycemia.

- Plan to monitor blood glucose at least four or more times a day — specifically, before meals and at bedtime. Your

Did You Know?
Diabetes Supplies at the Airport

It is always a good idea to alert airport security personnel if your child or teen is wearing an insulin pump and/ or carrying supplies that might be scanned. Diabetes supplies such as pens, syringes and meters can pass through scanners. As well, some insulin pumps can pass through metal detectors but not X-ray machines. Travelers whose pumps can't go through scanners will likely have to be patted down, which could require more time. (For more information, see Further Resources, "Travel and Diabetes.")

family's routine will be different than it is at home, and you'll need to know how the blood glucose levels are affected so you can make safe adjustments. A good rule of thumb during air travel across different time zones is to check blood glucose levels at least every four hours.

- For active holidays, you may need to reduce your child's insulin. Speak with members of your diabetes team ahead of time about how to plan for this.

- Make sure your child wears some form of diabetes identification, such as a medical-alert bracelet.

Q & A

Q. My 6-year-old son has been forgetting to eat his morning snack at school. He's been arriving home for lunch quite low some days. What should I do?

A. In general, 6-year-olds have no concept of time, and playing in the schoolyard often takes priority over eating a snack. It's unlikely your son is going to remember to take that snack on his own, and it's reasonable to expect your son's teacher to remind him when it's time. If the snack is interfering with play, consider something fast and easy to eat: for example, a few raisins instead of an apple. Or, if necessary, ask the teacher to give him the snack in class just prior to the recess break. If lows continue to occur, consider adjusting his insulin dose.

If a snack is interfering with play, consider something fast and easy to eat: for example, a few raisins instead of an apple.

Q. My son wants to go on a 10-day camping trip into the wilderness. He will be out of contact with civilization for most of the time. Should I let him go?

A. This is a decision for you and your son to make. Before agreeing to let him go, you should feel comfortable that he and his friends understand the issues involved in being out in the wilderness. Your son should have demonstrated good judgment and a high level of responsibility in diabetes care, and should be committed to doing more, rather than less, blood glucose testing on the trip.

You should make every effort to ensure that there is a way to be in touch with "civilization" if any urgent issues arise.

Q. My 11-year-old daughter has expressed interest in using the pump, but she is concerned that it may limit her participation in some of the sports she enjoys so much. Can she be active and still use an insulin pump?

A. Employing an insulin pump to manage her diabetes should not prevent your daughter from participating in most sports. The key elements to watch out for are protecting the insertion site, avoiding long, exposed lengths of catheter, and securing the pump so that it does not shake free during the sports activities. Some individuals choose sites for the catheter insertion that can easily be protected by their sports equipment or outfit. For some activities, an extra waistband under the uniform or equipment may successfully be used to secure the pump. Some pumps can be worn while swimming. Other children may disconnect the catheter from the infusion site for periods of about an hour during swim classes or competitions.

Q. How do I deal with a time-zone change?

A. There is no magic formula to help you figure out how to adjust insulin for a time-zone change — every situation and individual is different. Generally, if you will be traveling across more than three time zones, some type of insulin adjustment will be necessary. It is important to take into account the timing and duration of your different insulin doses, the length of your flights, the time-zone change and availability of food (you'll bring along extra, of course). Address these issues with your child's doctor or nurse, either at a clinic appointment or several weeks before you depart.

Those who are on insulin pump therapy or an MDI routine with long- and fast-acting insulin with food will find it much easier to deal with time-zone changes than those working with intermediate-acting insulins (Humulin-N, Novolin NPH). This being said, it is possible to make adjustments to any insulin routine so that you can get safely to your destination and make a switch to the new time zone in order to be doing everything (eating, sleeping, waking up) at the same time as the locals.

> Generally, if you will be traveling across more than three time zones, some type of insulin adjustment will be necessary.

HOW TO: Manage Insulin while Traveling Across Time Zones

Traveling East

Since traveling east will shorten your day, generally you will need to reduce the amount of long-acting insulin that your child usually takes. An example of this could be traveling from North America to Europe. You might depart in the evening and arrive at your destination seven hours later, in time for breakfast — having lost six to seven hours from your day. The departure time of your flight will have an impact on your child's or teen's long-acting insulin dose, and how much to decrease it, so make sure to discuss these important details with your diabetes team.

Traveling West

Since traveling west will lengthen your day, this means that your child will likely need more insulin and meals on the actual travel day. An example of this could be traveling from Europe to North America, during which you would gain an extra six to seven hours. Generally, this would mean that when your family arrives home, your child would need an extra meal and likely an extra dose of fast-acting insulin. By following this type of adjustment, you can often get back to your normal routines and start the next day as you usually would in terms of the timing of your diabetes care routines.

Q. Is it hard to get travel insurance?

A. As with life insurance and other forms of insurance, it can be more difficult for people with diabetes to obtain travel insurance. Your diabetes association may recommend specific travel insurers. You can also reach out to any other families you may know who have a child with diabetes to see what their experiences have been with traveling and obtaining coverage, if they don't have a plan through their work.

Chapter 11

The Diabetes Clinic Visit

After the initial stabilization at diagnosis, all those with type 1 diabetes are encouraged to attend the diabetes clinic *at least* three or four times every year for an assessment of their condition. In this chapter, we discuss how routine clinic visits play an essential role in good diabetes care.

Most of the time, these visits are like pit stops in a car race: a relatively quick check that the diabetes is in good control, with surveillance for both psychosocial and biomedical complications and any associated conditions seen more commonly with diabetes. These visits are excellent opportunities for you and your child or teen to have your concerns addressed, questions answered and plans laid out for special events and any upcoming anticipated changes.

Terminology

Psychosocial refers to the interrelation of social factors and individual behavior. *Biomedical* refers to factors that relate to both biology and medicine.

Key Messages

The routine clinic visit serves as an essential time:

- For the child or teen and family to have their concerns addressed
- For the diabetes team to assess the status of the diabetes and provide helpful advice and management
- To facilitate screening for complications and associated conditions

You will likely meet with more than one of your team members at this time or have a focused appointment with one health care professional. However, since over time most families are seen by multiple members of their health care team, it is crucial that important information is shared among team members and a joint plan of action generated. Many children and teens find it easier to talk to one team member in particular; however, children and teens need to be informed that their team functions as an integrated unit, with all members involved in supporting them and their family.

Occasionally at one of these appointments, the team discovers that there are a number of diabetes-related problems that need to be addressed in either more frequent follow-up appointments at clinic or with more planned time in the ambulatory setting not related to clinic (for example, a re-education session). Some problems can be resolved over the phone. Very occasionally, there is need for a hospital admission to sort out severe and difficult problems.

Research Spotlight

(Mis)communication

More than 30 years ago, a study was performed at a very large diabetes center in North America: children and teens with type 1 diabetes and their parents attending the clinic were seen by a pediatric endocrinologist (their diabetes doctor), a diabetes nurse and a dietitian. After the visit, each of the health care professionals was asked to list the three most important recommendations given to these families, while the families were asked to provide their own list of recommendations from each of the three health care professionals.

The result was totally unexpected: for most participants, there was simply no match between the lists provided by each of the health care professionals and those provided by the families. And this was immediately following the visit — not hours or days later. Clearly this study shows that the family and their care providers were not on the same page (attuned).

What to Expect at the Clinic Visit

Each clinic visit provides an opportunity to achieve some aspects of the following:

- A routine review of your child's or teen's progress, including: a review of blood glucose and insulin logs (or printouts); a discussion of any episodes of hypo-glycemia, intercurrent illness, school attendance and social adjustment; measurement of height and weight to assess growth; and the performance of an A1c test and other screening tests as indicated in the table in chapter 13.

- A discussion of what you and your child or teen wish to take from this clinic visit. Do you have specific questions about an upcoming school trip, for example, or about vaccinations? Make sure these questions are addressed directly before the end of the visit.

- A determination of what further steps are needed to ensure the ongoing achievement of treatment goals. The visit also allows the team to focus on important pieces of information that need to be reviewed or reinforced. The need to meet regularly with the diabetes dietitians is essential, since good nutritional practices are fundamental to achieving and maintaining good blood glucose control. As well, the nutritional plan will continuously evolve, since food intake is very much dependent on age, size, activity level and growth.

- A decision as to whether a young teen needs a more intensive review of their self-management. This may require an additional visit on another day.

- A review of the information from the pump and/or glucose meter, for a few reasons: first, to allow the diabetes team to get an overall view of patterns of blood glucose control; and second, to check up on the frequency with which both glucose testing and/or boluses have been missed. Missed blood glucose readings and skipped insulin injections are quite common causes of ongoing poor metabolic control.

- A chance to update prescriptions for diabetes supplies that will lessen the need for more calls between visits.

Psychosocial Evaluation

From the psychosocial standpoint, clinic visits allow team members to:

- Assess family stresses that could impact adherence to diabetes management, and make appropriate referrals to the mental health/behavioral specialists on the team.

- Ensure that developmentally appropriate family involvement is ongoing. Premature transfer of responsibility for diabetes care to the child or teen can result in nonadherence and deteriorating glucose control. Similarly, lack of appropriate teen involvement in self-care may be a source of ongoing conflict in the family.

- Spend time alone with adolescent patients. Starting at about 12 years of age, adolescents should have time alone with their health care providers in order to privately address their needs and to receive anticipatory guidance around issues such as conception and child-bearing, sexual activity (including contraception information) and sexuality, and alcohol and tobacco (smoking) or other substance use.

Physical Examination

From the standpoint of the physical examination, surveillance for complications includes:

- Measurement of height and weight: the expectation is that children and teens with type 1 diabetes will grow and develop in the same ways as their peers. Loss of weight suggests either poorly controlled diabetes or, in some teenagers, the onset of an eating disorder.

- Regular blood pressure measurements (twice yearly).

- Inspection of blood glucose monitoring and insulin injection or infusion sites. As noted previously, repeated insulin injection or pump infusion sites in the same area will lead to toughness of the area and deposition of fat at the site (called lipohypertrophy). Occasionally, loss of fat can also occur (**lipoatrophy**).

Additional aspects of the physical examination will be determined by symptoms or signs.

HOW TO: Get the Most out of the Diabetes Clinic Visit

Sometimes, the clinic visit seems to speed by very quickly and you may feel that you have not had your issues adequately addressed. There are a few things you and your child or teen can do ahead of time to make sure you get the most out of this visit.

Before the Clinic Visit

- Write out your questions and concerns so as not to forget them.
- Write down any recent symptoms of concern.
- Make sure you bring current self-monitoring records (blood glucose readings, insulin doses and changes) plus the glucose meter(s) and pump to the clinic visit.
- Know what the previous A1c level was.

After the Clinic Visit

- Make sure you have a list of recommendations to follow.
- Relay this information to those who were not at the clinic appointment so that there is consistency.
- Make sure you get the results of all tests performed or know how your doctor will follow up with you about any results.
- Make sure you have booked the next visit and have this marked in your calendar.

Surveillance for Associated Conditions

A sizeable proportion of people with type 1 diabetes, perhaps as many as one-third, will develop evidence of thyroid involvement. About 5% to 10% of people with type 1 diabetes will show evidence of antibodies to gluten.

Children and teens with type 1 diabetes are susceptible to specific comorbid conditions. In medicine, comorbidity is the presence of one or more additional diseases or conditions co-occurring with a primary disease or disorder. Two in particular, Hashimoto's thyroiditis (autoimmune thyroid disease) and celiac disease, are sufficiently frequent to warrant routine screening (see table in chapter 13). Like type 1 diabetes, these are also autoimmune disorders.

In addition, mental health issues such as depression, anxiety and adolescent adjustment are fairly frequent during the teen years and are known to be more common in those with type 1 diabetes or other chronic medical conditions.

Detailed information on surveillance for and early management of diabetes-related complications and comorbid conditions can be found in chapter 13.

Hashimoto's Thyroiditis/ Hypothyroidism

The **thyroid** sits at the base of the neck in front of the windpipe. Its role in humans is to secrete thyroxine, the hormone that sets the body's basal metabolic rate. Thyroid underactivity (hypothyroidism) slows down the body; thyroid overactivity (hyperthyroidism) speeds it up. A sizeable proportion of people with type 1 diabetes, perhaps as many as one-third, will develop evidence of thyroid involvement as noted by the presence in the blood of thyroid autoantibodies. Of these, some will develop enlargement of the thyroid gland, also called a **goiter**, and a smaller proportion will develop underactivity of the thyroid gland, either with no overt changes or in full-blown form.

Celiac Disease

Celiac disease is a result of an autoimmune reaction to gluten in the diet and leads to the loss of absorptive capacity of the bowels. Gluten is an integral part of wheats and related grains, including barley and rye. About 5% to 10% of those with type 1 diabetes will show evidence of antibodies to gluten when screened. Most will be asymptomatic. However, when a small bowel biopsy is performed, it's likely that doctors will find a flattening of the bowel lining, which decreases

CASE HISTORY
Celiac Symptoms

A 14-year-old girl was referred to us from a community pediatric diabetes unit because they were concerned about her poor growth over the past two years and about abdominal cramps and nausea that had been present for the past three months. She had a normal physical examination. Height and weight were both well below the third percentile, but no one had seemed concerned. A careful history-taking revealed that she had very smelly bowel movements that did not flush easily. A screening test revealed typical celiac antibodies, and a small bowel biopsy confirmed the diagnosis. She followed a fairly strict gluten-free diet and experienced a quick resolution of symptoms and good catch-up growth.

the absorptive capacity. Some will have symptoms including abdominal discomfort, cramps, diarrhea, poor weight gain and/or poor growth. When a gluten-free diet is introduced, the flattened villi in the bowel lining recover. There continues to be debate among physicians as to whether asymptomatic celiac disease calls for therapy with a gluten-free diet or not.

Mental Health Issues

The increased prevalence of mental health issues in children and teens with diabetes may be related generically to the presence of a lifelong medical condition with specific demands, or perhaps may be due to some increased likelihood of developing a mental health issue under such circumstances. Whichever is the case, there can be no doubt that the interaction between diabetes and mental health issues can severely test the ability to reach target glucose levels.

This demands the presence of team members trained in the behavioral specialties. These individuals can work with other team members to identify challenges early and intervene before they become more serious. Mental health professionals should be considered integral members of the interdisciplinary pediatric diabetes team.

Did You Know?
When to Ask for a Referral

Indications for referral to a mental health/behavioral specialist include:

- Repeated hospitalizations for DKA
- Significant distress
- School nonattendance/ refusal to attend
- Serious family dysfunction

The Role of the Family Doctor

Your relationship with your diabetes health care team cannot and should not replace the role of the family doctor or pediatrician in attending to your child's or teen's general health needs. Routine immunization, managing infections and annual physicals, if needed, should continue outside the diabetes team. Good communications should be established between the primary health care provider (family doctor or pediatrician) and the diabetes team so that your child or teen can avoid having tests duplicated or omitted.

Good communication is essential. Parents and diabetes specialists should keep the family doctor informed about the child's diabetes management plan. Likewise, the family doctor will communicate any concerns to the rest of the diabetes team.

Q & A

Q. My daughter gets quite anxious about her clinic visits as they get closer. Then she always seems to forget her glucose meter and logbook at home. What can I do to help?

A. It sounds as if your daughter is reluctant to have her diabetes team members learn that she is perhaps struggling with her diabetes management routines (for example, possibly missing blood glucose checks or forgetting to give boluses with her insulin pump). Forgetting to bring her meter, which would identify this, is one way of keeping this struggle private. Start by trying to have an honest conversation with your daughter about what might be causing her anxiety, and reinforce that she is part of a team that is there to help her try to achieve her diabetes care goals. Be sure to acknowledge how challenging it can be to fit all the demands of diabetes care into one's life, and ask what she thinks would be helpful for you and others to do to help her keep up with these management expectations.

Q. The other day, my son's diabetes doctor called him in on his own at the beginning of the appointment and asked me to join them only as they were wrapping up. This was the first time she had done this, and it made me feel excluded from the visit. Can I ask to be included in the full appointment at future visits?

A. Often, once children reach early adolescence, care providers do start to see teens on their own for part of their clinic visit. This is done for two reasons. First, it gives both the teen and the care provider a chance to discuss normal developmental topics that might be uncomfortable to discuss around parents. Second, it provides an opportunity for the teen to discuss their diabetes care independent of their parents, which is necessary as they get older and essential prior to their transition to adult care. You should absolutely be involved in the final part of your son's appointments to outline future goals, but encouraging your teen's independence by also allowing him to meet with his doctor on his own is appropriate.

Once children reach early adolescence, care providers do start to see teens on their own for part of their clinic visit.

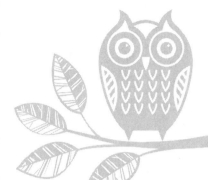

Chapter 12

Transition to Adult Care

There are many transitions that occur in the life of a child diagnosed with type 1 diabetes: from hospital to home with family members at the time of diagnosis; from starting daycare to being under the constant eye of the school personnel; from becoming an older school–age child with more freedom to entering early adolescence with increasing self-management.

All of these transitions have one thing in common: they usually take place with the full support of the family and pediatric (childhood) diabetes team. However, the final transition to an adult diabetes care center can be the most wrenching and, potentially, most difficult transition and adjustment of all. In this chapter, we focus attention on the transition from the children's center to the adult setting.

Key Messages

- Transition from child to adult diabetes care is a potentially stressful time.

- Preparation should include both formal and informal elements, and should start early.

- Transition should be an ongoing process and not something that occurs at one point in time.

- Close cooperation between the child/teen and adult centers is essential.

Transition to young adulthood can be incredibly challenging. It is almost always associated with a multitude of other changes — for instance, the completion of high school and start of postsecondary education, or entering the workforce. In addition, the young adult often leaves home at this time. In terms of diabetes care, this often means leaving the team at the children's hospital or in the children's section and moving to an adult facility.

This move to a new health care setting can be a similar experience to graduating from high school and moving away to college. Over a relatively short period of time, the teen shifts from being the biggest, oldest and wisest person to being a young, inexperienced "rookie" in a much larger, different and diverse environment. Some find the experience exciting; others prefer the comfort of their old setting.

CASE HISTORY
Parental Adjustment

Just before his 18th birthday, Jason came to the diabetes clinic with his dad for a final visit. The next clinic visit, three months ahead, had already been scheduled in the adult facility about two blocks away. Jason had completed informal and formal discussions regarding transition to the adult facility and what he should expect — such as attending the visits alone, rather than with his parents, and being expected to make follow-up visits and so on without the clinical personnel having to, well, "treat him like a child."

Jason was quite excited to be "getting out" of the children's hospital environment, where he had to share the waiting room with little kids. He left the office in good spirits. As he did, his dad asked to speak to the diabetes doctor for a few minutes. The doctor walked Jason to the waiting room, said goodbye and offered him his best wishes. He returned to his office to find Dad gently weeping: "How are we going to survive without our team?" he asked repeatedly. "You have always been available to help us through tricky situations. We depend on you guys."

Dad was told that he was welcome to contact the team until Jason was well set up in the adult center. He could call when he felt the need. He did so intermittently for a couple of months, until Jason was settled in at university and seeing the adult endocrinologist. The transition period allowed Dad to feel much better about the upheaval of leaving their "diabetes home."

The Process of Transition

Transition out of the clinic within the children's hospital to an adult facility — be it within a general hospital or in a community setting — is a pivotal event for young adults and their families, both of whom have grown used to the nurturing environment of the pediatric clinic. It is essential, therefore, that special and focused attention be paid to the process of transition. There are three aspects to the transition: preparation, separation and adaptation (or adoption).

- **Preparation:** Preparing for transition is not a single event that occurs just before the transfer to the adult facility. Rather, it begins at the time of diagnosis and continues throughout the child's or teen's time in the pediatric clinic: the whys and what to expect require reinforcement on many occasions.

- **Separation:** The date of the last visit should be arranged well in advance, and be looked upon as a chance for reinforcement of whys and wherefores, a chance to ensure follow-up is in place, and a chance, perhaps, for a few tears (on all sides!).

- **Adaptation/Adoption:** Pediatric diabetes centers should work with their adult counterparts to ensure as smooth a transition as possible. In our experience, the teens and their parents tend to feel supported leading up to the

Crossing the Rubicon

Some years ago, on Diabetes Day — our annual family education update — our team put on a short play dealing with an important scenario in diabetes care.

Act 1: Scene 1: Mom, Dad and teenage son are sitting in the waiting room of the children's hospital diabetes clinic for the last time. Dad is reading the newspaper, oblivious to the other two. Mom is extremely anxious, continuously stroking her son's head and saying how upset she is to leave the clinic. Their doctor walks into the waiting room and calls the family into his office for the last time.

Act 1: Scene 2: Dad continues to read his newspaper. The teen responds to a few questions but spends most of his time trying to brush his mom's hand away and get her to stop asking so many questions. Repeatedly he says: I know all this… The scene ends with a teary goodbye.

Act 2: Scene 1: The teen and Mom are sitting quietly among a group of older people in the adult endocrinologist's office. Mom is agitated, trying to hide her anxiety, but not succeeding. The doctor arrives, calls in the son and asks Mom to wait in the waiting room (they had been warned that this would happen). Mom asks if she can't come in, just this once. Both the doctor and son say no, quite forcefully. As the doctor and son turn to walk into the office, Mom grabs hold of her son's leg and is dragged along behind him. Seeing this, the doctor hauls out a cell phone and says: "Houston, we have a problem!!" echoing the astronauts detecting a serious problem during the aborted moonflight of *Apollo 13.*

The scene is, for effect, a little melodramatic, but it does suggest that Mom is ill-prepared for this change. It also suggests that Mom has not yet "let go" sufficiently to let her son take over the 100% of diabetes care that is now his. More support from Dad may also have made things somewhat easier.

transfer. At this point, however, they may experience some discomfort around the changes from a family-centered to patient-centered approach to care. For many teens and parents, this may be a difficult and giant leap rather than a small step. Knowing what to expect during and after the transition can make this an easier time for the family, as can efforts to gradually increase the teen's "ownership" of their diabetes care. (See "How to Support Transition Long Before the Actual Transfer to Adult Care" on page 191, for more information.)

> Knowing what to expect during and after the transition can make this an easier time for the family, as can efforts to gradually increase the teen's "ownership" of their diabetes care.

The Impact of Transition on the Teen and Parents

The figure below is a modification of a model of life transitions developed in the 1970s by psychologists Barrie Hopson and John Adams. In it, the impacts of the transition process on the teen and parents are shown as two very different paths at the point of moving from pediatric to adult care. The hope is that they will meet again over time as ongoing stable care is established.

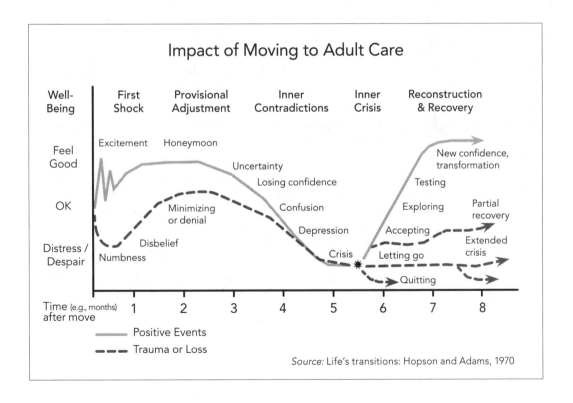

After a period of perhaps unrealistic optimism, there is often a period of uncertainty and confusion for the emerging young adult.

Our interpretation of this model is that the solid line represents the adolescent, feeling relatively good about themselves at the point of transition to adult care. Unfortunately, the parents, represented by the broken line, are much less happy about moving into a new and unknown environment of health care for their child. The model does suggest that, after a period of perhaps unrealistic optimism, there is often a period of uncertainty and confusion for the emerging young adult. Often, the new demands of adult care and emphasis on complications screening can be overwhelming, and the newly graduated teenager can feel incapable of meeting them. Some young adults are tempted to drop out of care altogether.

Did You Know?

Transition Programs

It is helpful for a teen leaving the pediatric center to take part in either an individual or group program that stresses the need for ongoing excellent blood glucose control, surveillance for complications, and changing expectations.

Making a Successful Transition

How well the transfer is navigated will depend on the individual young adult and the new team involved in their care. As well, the support of family and friends throughout the transition phase is vital to ensure that the young adult continues with the care needed to manage their diabetes.

Ideally, the change to adult care should come when the teenager is confident and responsible enough to move forward. Unfortunately, hospital or clinic policy usually dictates a transition between the ages of 16 and 20. Parents and teens should be aware of this well ahead of time in order to prepare.

Parents can help teens make a successful transfer by encouraging them to take an active part in their diabetes care throughout childhood and adolescence. When parents encourage their children to problem-solve and make choices about adjusting insulin doses, for example, they set the foundation for the self-management behaviors that are essential in adulthood. Teenagers also need private time with all members of the diabetes team, as this promotes independence and responsibility. Before being discharged from the pediatric center, teens should have the opportunity to explore various options for continuing their diabetes health care, and a referral should be made to the adult team.

HOW TO: Support Transition Long Before the Actual Transfer to Adult Care

- Encourage your teen to see their physician and other team members privately for at least part of each clinic appointment.

- Let your teen speak and answer questions.

- Involve and empower your teen in management decisions (for example, insulin dose changes).

- Encourage your teen to directly contact diabetes team members with questions or to report on how things are going.

- Ask your teen to determine one or two things that they'd like to "get out" of their clinic appointment prior to the visit.

- Help your teen anticipate and problem-solve certain situations that could come up around their diabetes care (for example, forgetting to take insulin when they go out).

- Help your teen identify friends that could be helpful and ways they could be positively involved.

- Attend transition programs offered by your local diabetes center.

Q & A

Q. After my daughter "graduates" from the diabetes clinic at the hospital, is it okay for her to be seen just by her family doctor?

A. It's still important for your daughter to have access to all members of the diabetes health care team (doctor, nurse, dietitian, social worker), even after she leaves the children's clinic. There are obstacles to navigate at each age and stage of development, such as moving away to college or university, living on her own, changes in exercise or activity patterns, frequent trips away from home on business — the list goes on and on. These are best dealt with by health care professionals experienced in diabetes care. If your family doctor is one of these, then he or she may well meet your daughter's needs.

Q. My daughter and I are both concerned that she will not get along with her new doctor as well as she did with her pediatric doctor. Who should we turn to if things are not going well at the new center?

A. It often takes a little while, perhaps three or four visits, before teens start to feel "at home" in the adult center. Keep this in mind, and try not to jump to quick conclusions about how the new setup may or may not work for you or your teen. Make sure you attend all of your clinic visits, and come prepared with blood glucose logs and pump printouts. If after some time the fit is just not there, contact the team at the children's center for an alternate referral.

> It often takes a little while, perhaps three or four visits, before teens start to feel "at home" in the adult center.

Q. When my child transitions to their new adult diabetes doctor, will I, as the parent, still be able to come to the appointments?

A. While attending the initial appointments with your teen may provide important support in the new environment, part of the process of adolescents becoming more independent with their diabetes care is for them to start attending appointments alone. To aid in this transition, it can be helpful if your child spends some time during their pediatric diabetes appointments alone with their team. This gives them the opportunity to "practice" independence prior to transitioning to adult care.

Q. Are there ways I can help prepare my child for her eventual move to adult care?

A. Yes! Supporting your teen through all of the normal developmental transitions that precede the move to adult care is imperative in order for them to be fully prepared. You can do this by empowering them to incorporate their diabetes management into settings when they are on their own with their peers (perhaps on school trips or during sleepovers). You can also help them to gradually become more informed about and involved in specific aspects of their care, such as making insulin dose changes and contacting members of their team directly, as needed. Having your teen participate in booking their follow-up appointments and letting you know when they are running low on their supplies is also important practice for when they will manage these aspects of their care more independently.

Chapter 13

Putting Complications in Perspective

After the discovery of insulin in 1921, diabetes was no longer immediately life-threatening. Doctors expected that all the problems of the disease would also disappear. Unfortunately, this was not the case, and it soon was recognized that long-term high blood glucose levels can be associated with the development of specific diabetes-related complications. In this chapter, we address the complications of diabetes, their detection, prevention and management, as well as associated conditions found together with type 1 diabetes.

Key Messages

- The rate of complications in type 1 diabetes has decreased significantly over the past 20 to 30 years as a result of more children and teens achieving tighter blood glucose control.

- It is important to perform regular screening for signs of diabetes-related complications so that they can be detected at an early and potentially reversible stage.

- Optimizing diabetes control to lower the A1c to target is the most effective way to reduce the risk for the onset and/or progression of long-term complications.

Over the last several decades, researchers have learned a great deal about these complications, their symptoms, causes and treatment, and how to slow their progression. Perhaps most important, researchers are now devising ways to prevent complications altogether.

We know, however, that maintaining optimal diabetes control is hard work and, because obvious complications are very rare in young people, the threat of developing these

....

There is no absolute level of blood glucose control or A1c that separates those who will develop long-term complications from those who will not.

....

complications is rarely a motivator. Most young people seldom think about their health 20 years down the road, and children with diabetes are no exception. That's where parents, family members and health care professionals come in — to provide the foresight and support to help them stay on track toward a healthy future.

What Are the Complications of Diabetes?

The physical long-term diabetes-related complications fall into two groups: microvascular (involving the small blood vessels of the body) and macrovascular (involving large blood vessels). While microvascular complications occur only in people with diabetes, macrovascular complications also occur in the general population, but to a lesser extent.

Microvascular complications include:

- Retinopathy, or eye damage
- Nephropathy, or kidney damage
- Neuropathy, or nerve damage

Macrovascular complications include:

- Cardiovascular disease, or risk of heart attack
- Cerebrovascular disease, or risk of stroke
- Peripheral vascular disease, or poor circulation to the limbs, which may cause foot problems and may lead to amputation

It is important to emphasize that not everyone with diabetes will develop any or all of these problems. Furthermore, there is no absolute level of blood glucose control or A1c that separates those who will develop long-term complications from those who will not.

Long-term diabetes-related complications are extremely rare in young children and uncommon during the teenage years. However, diabetes probably has effects from the time of onset. The impact may be somewhat less before puberty, but early changes seem to accelerate during the teenage years. Indeed, follow-up studies from the Diabetes Control and Complications Trial showed that diabetes control in the teenage years is especially important in determining long-term complication risk as an adult. This concept, known as metabolic memory, strongly suggests that efforts to maintain good blood glucose balance should begin right from the time of diagnosis of the diabetes.

Research Spotlight

Preventing Complications

The best way to prevent complications from diabetes is to maintain blood glucose control as close to normal as possible. A very important research study performed in the 1980s and 1990s, called the Diabetes Control and Complications Trial, demonstrated that lower average blood glucose levels and A1c are associated with a significant decreased risk in the chance of developing long-term diabetes-related complications. Those patients in the trial who were in the group with lower A1c levels had between a 50% and 75% reduced risk of developing eye, kidney or nerve complications. Even in those patients who were unable to achieve target A1c levels, every 1% reduction in their A1c was associated with a 30% reduced risk of diabetes-related eye complications.

The long-term follow up of the patients in this study, the Epidemiology of Diabetes Interventions and Complications, continues to demonstrate benefits of tighter blood glucose control on both small and large blood vessel complications.

Risk Factors for Diabetes-Related Complications

Some risk factors, such as duration of diabetes, cannot be changed, while others, including glucose control, can.

- **Duration of diabetes:** Even the very earliest stages of these complications are rare in those who have had type 1 diabetes for less than five years, and before the onset of puberty. After that, the longer a person has had diabetes, the more likely it is that complications will arise.

- **Suboptimal blood glucose control:** The Diabetes Control and Complications Trial clearly demonstrated that blood glucose control counts. Independent of any other risk factors, such as high blood pressure or being overweight, excellent blood glucose control decreases the development of complications. However, that doesn't mean that someone with poor control is guaranteed to have complications, and nor does it mean that someone with excellent control is guaranteed not to have them.

- **Smoking:** Many studies show that tobacco smokers with diabetes are at much greater risk of developing complications, and that these complications worsen

> Independent of any other risk factors, such as high blood pressure or being overweight, excellent blood glucose control decreases the development of complications.

more rapidly when compared to nonsmokers. Giving up smoking decreases the risk considerably. It is best never to start smoking in the first place. Nonetheless, successful cessation of smoking will decrease ongoing risk substantially.

- **High blood pressure:** People with diabetes who develop high blood pressure (hypertension) are at high risk of complications because of increased pressure on the kidneys, heart and blood vessels. Lowering the blood pressure with medical treatment reduces this risk. Regular blood pressure checks allow early detection of hypertension. Aggressive control of blood pressure will lessen the risk of complication development or progression.

- **High blood fats:** People with poor blood glucose control are more likely to develop high blood fat (**lipid**) levels (**hyperlipidemia**), including high cholesterol and high triglycerides. There are also people who are born with a tendency to develop high blood fat levels. In both cases, these high levels contribute to the risk of complications.

- **Obesity:** People who are overweight are at increased risk for macrovascular complications. Weight control may be a difficult challenge for teens and adults, especially girls, who are much more likely than boys to develop an eating disorder in response to repeated efforts to control weight.

Screening for Complications and Associated Conditions

It is very unusual for children before the onset of puberty, or those who have had type 1 diabetes for less than three to five years, to show evidence of long-term complications. Even in teens who have had type 1 diabetes for five or ten years, advanced complications are extremely unusual. Nevertheless, once puberty has started and diabetes has been present for three to five years, screening for complications and risk factors should begin.

In youth with type 2 diabetes, complications can start earlier, even from the time of diagnosis. Screening for these complications needs to therefore also start much earlier.

In both type 1 and 2 diabetes, it's reassuring when no problems are found. But if the early stages of complications are detected, it allows intervention to occur at a stage when the changes are potentially reversible or at least can be slowed down.

Here are some of the blood and urine tests and examinations that your diabetes team will recommend on a regular basis. More frequent testing will likely be advised if any abnormalities are discovered.

Complication/ Condition	Frequency of Screening in Type 1 Diabetes	Frequency of Screening in Type 2 Diabetes	Screening Method
Hypertension (high blood pressure)	At least twice a year	At diagnosis and at least twice a year	Measure blood pressure using an appropriate-sized blood pressure cuff
Hyperlipidemia (high blood fats)	At 12 and 17 years of age In those <12 years, screen if extra risk factors (obesity/family history of hyperlipidemia/early onset cardiovascular disease)	At diagnosis and then every 1 to 3 years	Blood test done while the child is fasting, assessing cholesterol (total, HDL and LDL) and triglyceride levels
Retinopathy (eye-related diabetes complications)	Once a year after the teen is 15 years of age and has had diabetes for more than 5 years	Once a year from diagnosis	Optometrist or ophthalmologist looks at or photographs the blood vessels at the back of the eye
Nephropathy (kidney-related diabetes complications)	Once a year after the teen is 12 years of age and has had diabetes for more than 5 years	Once a year from diagnosis	Urine sample for the albumin/creatinine ratio (the amount of protein in the urine) First morning urine sample is preferred
Neuropathy (nerve-related diabetes complications)	Once a year in teenagers with poor diabetes control who have completed puberty and have had diabetes for at least 5 years	Once a year from diagnosis	Diabetes team to ask and examine for symptoms of numbness, pain, altered sensation in the feet or toes and reduced ankle tendon reflexes
Hashimoto's thyroiditis/ hypothyroidism (autoimmune thyroid disease)	At diagnosis and every 2 years thereafter Every 6 to 12 months in children with a large thyroid gland or evidence of thyroid antibodies on blood testing	Not needed	Blood test for thyroid hormone level (thyroid stimulating hormone — TSH) and thyroid antibody level (thyroperoxidase antibodies — TPO)
Celiac disease	If there are symptoms such as abdominal pain, altered bowel habits, unexpected low blood glucose readings, poor growth or weight changes	Not needed	Blood test for the antibody associated with celiac disease (tissue transglutaminase) plus immunoglobulin A levels
Addison's disease (autoimmune adrenal disease)	If there are indicators of unexpected low blood glucose readings and reduced insulin doses	Not needed	Morning (8 a.m.) blood test for cortisol (an adrenal hormone), sodium and potassium

Diabetic Retinopathy

Diabetic retinopathy occurs when there is damage to the retina, the light-sensitive lining at the back of the eyeball. The condition has a slow progression, with changes seen only on careful examination of the eye by an experienced optometrist or **ophthalmologist** (health care providers who specialize in eye care) or through taking photographs of the retina. In its early and even late stages, retinopathy does not usually interfere with vision. Once vision loss begins, it suggests that the retinopathy is advanced.

The earliest changes are called background (non-proliferative) retinopathy and consist of little swellings of the blood vessels, called microaneurysms, which may start to leak or burst, causing leaking (exudates) and bleeding (hemorrhages). Vision is only compromised if the bleeding affects the part of the eye that focuses on the object of vision (the **macula**) or if that area swells (macular edema). Most patients with type 1 diabetes will develop background retinopathy after having the disease for 15 to 20 years.

This early stage of retinopathy may progress to proliferative retinopathy, where the eye begins to make new blood vessels to provide better blood flow. These new vessels are fragile and may cause bleeding and scarring in the fluid chamber (vitreous body) in front of the retina. The scarring, due to the bleeding, can cause the retina to separate or pull away from the eye; this is called retinal detachment. Proliferative retinopathy and its consequences are a major cause of partial or complete loss of sight. However, this does not mean that most people with diabetes will lose their vision.

Researchers have made great strides in repairing vision and reducing the risk of blindness in people with diabetes. Photocoagulation is a laser therapy technique that prevents blindness by destroying abnormal blood vessels, repairing leaking ones and stopping new ones from forming. This should reduce the risk of blindness by more than 75% to 80%. Occasionally, if the retina has bled too much or has become detached, surgery may be required. New medications are also being used to treat diabetic eye disease.

Regular screening for retinopathy will allow timely intervention and markedly reduce the risk of visual impairment or blindness.

Diabetic Nephropathy

The kidneys are the body's filtering system to remove waste products. As blood flows through the blood vessels into the kidneys, toxins and waste are removed and transported out of the kidneys, and out of the body, in the urine.

The relationship between diabetes and kidney disease is complex. Kidneys may enlarge and become overworked, resulting in a condition called diabetic nephropathy.

Not all people with type 1 diabetes develop nephropathy. It is more likely to occur after puberty, in people who have had type 1 diabetes for 15 years or longer. Poor blood glucose control, high blood pressure and smoking (or chewing) tobacco also increase the risk of kidney disease.

Signs and Symptoms: Nephropathy

Nephropathy, like retinopathy, develops slowly and quietly, with no symptoms or signs until serious kidney damage has occurred. Symptoms and signs may include:

- Higher blood pressure than usual
- Puffy ankles due to water retention (edema)
- Excessive protein in the urine (proteinuria)

Diabetic nephropathy can be detected at a very early stage, before it causes symptoms. This early phase is marked by the presence of very small amounts of a protein called albumin in the urine. This is called **microalbuminuria**; it can be detected in a first-morning or random urine specimen. If nephropathy progresses, the amount of protein in the urine will steadily increase to the stage of **overt proteinuria**. At this stage, protein can be detected by means of a routine dipstick of the urine.

Did You Know?
Preventing Nephropathy or Slowing Progression

Recent research has demonstrated that the onset of diabetic nephropathy can be prevented, or its progression significantly slowed, by achieving and maintaining excellent blood glucose control. Further progression can also be prevented or slowed with specific medications, such as certain blood pressure medications, called **angiotensin converting enzyme (ACE) inhibitors** or angiotensin II receptor blockers (ARBs). New groups of medications are also being tried to help prevent the progression of microalbuminuria.

If nephropathy remains untreated, it can progress to chronic renal (kidney) failure and eventually to end-stage renal failure, which requires dialysis or transplantation. Advanced nephropathy is also associated with a significant increased risk of macrovascular (large blood vessel) complications and early death due to diabetes. Because of this, early detection and treatment are essential to help optimize long-term health.

Diabetic Neuropathy

High blood glucose levels over the long term can also affect the nerves in many areas of the body. Some slowing of the electrical impulses that travel along the nerves is common in people with diabetes. However, some people go on to develop symptoms and signs of more severe neuropathy. This is extremely rare in children and teens.

Signs and Symptoms: Neuropathy

Neuropathy commonly affects the nerves to the arms and the legs and is characterized by:

- Tingling in the fingers and toes, extending toward the body
- Numbness (loss of feeling) in these areas
- Painful burning or freezing sensations, particularly in the feet
- Cramping or weakness
- Inability to detect hot and cold temperatures

Autonomic neuropathy, which is very unusual in childhood or adolescence, affects the nerves that go to internal organs, such as the gastrointestinal system or bladder. When the gastrointestinal system is affected, there may be problems with the stomach (including vomiting and difficulty moving the food into the intestines, along with bloating, called gastroparesis) or with the intestines (including constipation or, more commonly, diarrhea). Therapy is difficult, but may include smaller meal sizes and medications to improve intestinal action.

Nerve damage affecting the bladder can lead to urine retention or loss of bladder control. In some cases, men experience sexual dysfunction or impotence. These problems can be improved significantly with better blood glucose control and, if needed, medication.

Pro Tip

Symptoms of neuropathy can come and go, and are influenced by the level of blood glucose control. Certain prescription medications may alleviate the pain.

Foot Problems

The risk of foot problems as a complication of diabetes in children and adolescents is extremely low. As people with diabetes get older, they are more susceptible to infections and slow healing, due to poor circulation and the effects of diabetic neuropathy. A person with neuropathy can get a cut on the sole of the foot, or a blister from an ill-fitting shoe, and not even know it. This is especially likely to happen if the injury is the first indicator of neuropathy and the feet are not being examined each day. If the cut remains unnoticed, it can quickly become infected and, in the worst case, lead to gangrene (tissue death).

Although children don't usually experience foot infections, poor healing or gangrene, it's wise for them to develop good foot care habits so that problems can be avoided as they get older. From an early age, they should be taught how to take good care of their feet, just as they learn how to take good care of their hair, teeth and other parts of their body. Good foot care means keeping the feet clean and dry, wearing proper-fitting shoes, cutting toenails straight across rather than rounding them, avoiding ingrown toenails, and getting into the habit of examining the feet for cuts and blisters on a regular basis.

Macrovascular Complications

As people age, so do their large blood vessels. The term for this aging process is arteriosclerosis (often called hardening of the arteries). People with type 1 diabetes are susceptible to early aging of their large blood vessels, as are people who smoke, are obese, have persistently high blood fats or have uncontrolled high blood pressure. Arteriosclerosis can lead to heart attacks or heart failure (cardiovascular disease), strokes (cerebrovascular disease) or foot problems (peripheral vascular disease). As in other complications of diabetes, the risk can be reduced by maintaining excellent blood glucose control, keeping blood pressure in check, exercising regularly, eating a healthy diet and not smoking.

Pro Tip

Macrovascular complications are an ominous sign. Fortunately, they are almost unheard of in teens.

Other Medical Conditions

Type 1 diabetes is an autoimmune condition in which the body's immune system attacks and destroys the insulin–producing cells. There are a number of other autoimmune conditions known to be more commonly seen in children with type 1 diabetes. The three most common are hypothyroidism (underactive thyroid gland), celiac disease (intolerance to gluten) and Addison's disease (underactive adrenal gland). This does not mean that every child, or even most children, with type 1 diabetes will develop these other conditions, but as they can be more commonly seen, they are routinely screened for.

Youth with type 2 diabetes are not at increased risk for these autoimmune conditions. They do, however, have an increased risk for the development of fatty liver disease or, in girls, polycystic ovarian syndrome (see chapter 6 for more details).

Hashimoto's Thyroiditis/Hypothyroidism (Autoimmune Thyroid Disease)

The thyroid is a gland in the neck that produces thyroid hormone. Thyroid hormone is an important regulator for many metabolic processes in the body, such as growth, digestion, body temperature, weight and mood. Children with type 1 diabetes are most commonly at increased risk of developing underactive thyroid disease (hypothyroidism) because of the development of antibodies that affect the cells producing the thyroid hormone.

Signs and Symptoms: Hypothyroidism

- Goiter — enlargement of the thyroid gland
- Decreased growth
- Weight gain
- Feeling more tired
- Dry skin or hair
- Constipation
- Feeling the cold more than other people
- Problems concentrating

Screening for hypothyroidism includes regular blood tests to assess the level of TSH — thyroid stimulating hormone — and measure the antibodies that can work against the thyroid gland (TPO — thyroperoxidase antibodies). If hypothyroidism does develop, the treatment consists of taking synthetic thyroid hormone, called levothyroxine, in pill form.

Very rarely, children with type 1 diabetes can develop autoimmune overactive thyroid disease, called hyperthyroidism or Graves' disease. Hyperthyroidism can be treated in a variety of different ways, including using medication.

Signs and Symptoms: Hyperthyroidism

- Weight loss
- Increased appetite
- Sweating and often feeling hot
- Mood swings and agitation
- Diarrhea
- Bulging eyes

Celiac Disease

Celiac disease is a condition in which the body develops a sensitivity to gluten; it is seen more frequently in children with type 1 diabetes than in the general population. Gluten is a protein found in wheat, rye and barley. Intolerance to gluten damages the lining of the small intestine, making it harder for nutrients to be absorbed. Celiac disease can also interfere with diabetes control, as it can affect the ability of the body to absorb carbohydrate in the food. This can lead to unexplained low blood glucose levels (hypoglycemia).

In children with symptoms that may be related to celiac disease, screening is done by taking a blood test to look for certain antibodies (tissue transglutaminase antibodies — anti-tTG antibodies). Some diabetes clinics may regularly screen for celiac disease in all patients. If the blood test is positive, the child will be referred to a gastroenterologist (intestine specialist) to see if further testing is needed. This may include using a camera (endoscopy) while they are anaesthetized (asleep) to obtain a sample, or biopsy, of the lining of the small intestine. This is needed to confirm the diagnosis.

The treatment of celiac disease involves avoiding all gluten-containing foods as well as other potential gluten sources in the environment (such as some types of makeup or creams). A dietitian can help to educate the family about what changes to the diet are needed to safely achieve this. There are many naturally gluten-free foods, such as rice, corn and some ancient grains, and a wide variety of gluten-free options in regular supermarkets, specialty food shops and restaurants.

> ### Did You Know?
> **Symptoms of Celiac Disease**
>
> Many children with type 1 diabetes have no symptoms of celiac disease. Some children may experience abdominal bloating or pain, diarrhea, foul-smelling stools, poor growth or weight changes.

Examples of Gluten-Containing Foods and Sources

Grain Products

- Bread, pasta, cereals or baked goods made from wheat, rye or barley
- Couscous

Sources of "Hidden" Gluten

- Soups
- Salad dressings

- Ice cream
- Hotdogs and sausage
- Energy bars and trail mix

Environmental Sources

- Shampoos
- Cosmetics
- Medications
- Vitamins and supplements
- Lipsticks and lip balms

Addison's Disease

Addison's disease is a condition in which there is autoimmune destruction of the adrenal glands. The adrenal glands normally produce important hormones in the body — including the "stress hormone" cortisol and a hormone that helps to regulate the salt levels in the body, called aldosterone. In Addison's disease, the body stops producing enough of these hormones, which can lead to symptoms including tiredness, weight loss, vomiting and increased low blood glucose levels, or hypoglycemia. If not treated, Addison's can, over time, lead to severe illness, including shock. While Addison's disease is more common in children with type 1 diabetes than in the general population, it is still very rare, and much less frequent than autoimmune thyroid or celiac disease. Addison's disease can be diagnosed via a blood test and treated with oral medication.

Q & A

Q. Is it all right for my 6-year-old daughter with diabetes to go barefoot at the beach?

A. If you think it is safe for anyone in your family to walk around with bare feet on the beach, then it should be safe for your daughter too. A child with diabetes will have no more trouble healing than other members of the family.

Q. Is my child more likely to need glasses because of the diabetes?

A. Children with diabetes are no more likely than their nondiabetic friends to need glasses for either near- or far-sightedness. Diabetes does not cause permanent problems with vision unless retinopathy has become severe. This is exceptionally rare during childhood and adolescence. Sometimes, rapid changes in blood glucose can cause changes to the lens of the eye: swelling (if the glucose is very high) or contraction (if the glucose is very low). This can cause temporary blurring of vision. Balancing the blood glucose will invariably correct this. Nevertheless, a child who complains of difficulty seeing the chalkboard, or who has to sit close to the television, should have an eye exam to see if glasses are required. This is the same as in any child without diabetes.

Q. My teenage daughter has type 1 diabetes. So far, her doctor has not recommended any special eye or kidney tests. Is this okay?

A. It may be that your doctor has not initiated these checks because your daughter has had diabetes for less than five years. Regular screening should start after the onset of puberty and should also be done for children who have had diabetes longer than five years. If your daughter has had diabetes for that long, don't hesitate to bring up your concerns with your doctor; ask for a referral to an ophthalmologist (eye specialist) and request a urine check for microalbuminuria.

Q. Does having diabetes mean that my child is more likely to develop kidney or bladder infections?

A. Poorly controlled diabetes with very high glucose readings may lead to an increased susceptibility to bladder or vaginal infections. Diabetic nephropathy (kidney damage) does not cause an increased risk of kidney or bladder infection.

Q. Do oral contraceptives increase the risk of diabetes-related complications?

A. Research shows that women with diabetes (but no other risk factors) who use the contraceptive pill are not at any greater risk of complications than those who use other forms of contraception. The pills used today have much lower dosages of estrogen (the female hormone) than previous versions.

Q. I have heard that impotence is a complication of diabetes in men. Is this true?

A. Some men do experience impotence as a complication of long-duration diabetes. This may be the result of nerve damage and circulation problems associated with long-standing diabetes and inadequate blood glucose control. Careful attention to diabetes self-management and blood glucose control is the best way to stay healthy and prevent impotence.

Did You Know?
Smoking

There is a lot of research to show that people with diabetes who choose to smoke are at greater risk for developing both microvascular and macrovascular complications. Also, they are likely to take more time off work or school when they have minor illnesses such as a cold or flu.

Chapter 14

Current and Evolving Therapies for Diabetes

Since the discovery of insulin, important steps and even leaps have been made in understanding the cause, course and treatment of both type 1 and type 2 diabetes. However, despite this, only some of these advances have led to significant changes in the lives of those with diabetes.

In this chapter we will discuss some of the more recent advances, particularly technological advances, that have made significant changes in how we can manage diabetes, as well as research advances in understanding the cause and potential cure for diabetes in the future.

A cure may be more elusive than the optimists or the media would have us believe.

Key Messages

- Over the past 90-plus years, there have been significant advances in the understanding and management of diabetes, with ongoing research that promises even greater therapeutic advances in the years ahead.

- Recent advances have led to new ways of giving insulin, monitoring blood glucose levels, and detecting and treating complications, and may one day lead to different therapies that could cure diabetes.

- Technological advances hold enormous promise for the future development of an artificial pancreas.

Advances in research usually take many years to move through the appropriate stages of testing: first in test tubes, then in animals, and finally in people. Sometimes, research that initially seems successful doesn't work out in the long run. While it's disappointing that these experiments don't always lead to new treatment approaches, this work often advances our understanding of diabetes in important ways.

Some people with diabetes (as well as those with other conditions) are quite skeptical, believing that the research and medical communities have the ability to cure their disease, but refrain from doing so because there is too much profit to be made. Nothing could be further from the truth. Both type 1 and type 2 diabetes pose a massive public health burden worldwide. It has been suggested that more than 10% of all health care dollars are related in some way to diabetes. A cure is in everyone's best interests. However, a cure may be more elusive than the optimists or the media would have us believe.

Advances in Diabetes Management

Although the basic treatment of type 1 diabetes has changed little over the past 75 years in terms of the need for insulin administration, major advances have been made in a number of areas.

- The variety and purity of insulin preparations, and methods for delivering insulin under the skin, such as insulin pens and pumps
- New and ever-improving methods for monitoring blood glucose and other measures of blood glucose control, such as the A1c test
- The team approach and other methods of lifestyle management to help prevent psychosocial and long-term physical side effects

Insulin

For many years, the only insulins available were relatively impure preparations of beef and pork insulin. While these were effective in controlling blood glucose levels, they were sometimes associated with side effects such as insulin allergy, lipoatrophy or lipohypertrophy. Over the past 30 years, we have progressed through the development of highly purified pork insulin, to the availability of genetically engineered human insulins, to the recent production of insulin analogs — insulins that have been chemically or genetically altered to change their action time. For example, fast-acting insulins such as lispro or aspart are quicker in onset, higher in peak and shorter in duration than human insulin. In addition to the fast-acting insulins, there are also relatively "peakless" long-acting insulins such as glargine (Lantus) and detemir (Levemir). There are also even newer insulin preparations in various stages of development, including even faster-acting forms.

Did You Know?

Don't Rush to Judgment

View the latest news item or recent social-media post with a critical eye, and get as much information as you can from health care professionals, diabetes journals and other sources before forming an opinion.

Insulin Delivery Systems

Insulin pens have made insulin injections less painful and more convenient. The needles are shorter, finer and less painful, but are as reliable as the bigger needles. Smaller and more reliable insulin infusion pumps have also been developed. Pumps don't eliminate the need for a needle or for careful attention to blood glucose control, but they do allow for flexibility in the timing and amounts of meals eaten without compromising safety or control. Pumps are meeting with increasing enthusiasm among children and teens.

> There have been significant improvements in blood glucose monitoring systems, with the development of smaller, more reliable, user-friendly meters with enhanced memory systems, as well as easier-to-use finger-pricking devices.

Blood Glucose Monitoring

In the late 1970s, blood glucose monitoring began to replace urine glucose testing — a major advance in diabetes management. In the years since, there have been significant improvements in monitoring systems, with the development of smaller, more reliable, user-friendly meters with enhanced memory systems, as well as easier-to-use finger-pricking devices. Information in most blood glucose meters can now be uploaded to your computer or phone to allow for easier tracking of blood glucose levels and identification of patterns to help with dosing changes.

Despite all of these different options, making the time on an ongoing basis to review this information, identify blood glucose trends and change insulin dosing continues to be an essential part of optimizing diabetes care.

Continuous Glucose Monitoring

Continuous glucose monitoring (often called CGM) is a tool that allows frequent blood glucose checks, including information about the directional trend of the glucose values, without having to poke your finger. Glucose levels are instead measured every five minutes using a sensor that sits just underneath the skin.

Like any new technology, there are potential advantages — but there are also disadvantages that need to be considered when deciding whether CGM is going to work for your child. In addition, it is always important to remember that CGM does not completely replace the role of finger-poke blood glucose monitoring, as there are several situations in which this may still need to be done.

How Does CGM Work?

While there are different brands of CGM on the market that continue to be updated, and more are in development, they all consist of three distinct parts:

1. **Sensor:** The sensor is a very fine electrode that sits just underneath the skin. It measures the blood glucose in the fluid surrounding the cells underneath the skin (the interstitial fluid). The sensor is embedded using a special device that contains a small needle. The needle inserts the sensor but is then withdrawn. Depending on the CGM device, the sensor can be worn in the same locations where insulin injections are given and needs to be replaced every 6 to 14 days.

2. **Transmitter:** The transmitter attaches to the top of the sensor; it is what sits on top of the skin. It sends the blood glucose information to the receiver wirelessly.

3. **Receiver:** The receiver displays and stores the blood glucose information that is collected from the sensor and sent via the transmitter. The type of receiver varies depending on the CGM system being used. For some systems, the receiver is the child's insulin pump. In other systems, the blood glucose levels are sent to an app on a mobile phone or to a separate receiver device. All receivers display information on the current blood glucose level and the direction the blood glucose is moving (that is, whether it is increasing, decreasing or staying the same), and show a graphical display of how the blood glucose levels have been trending over the past several hours.

Some of the CGM devices also require blood glucose calibrations to be entered into the receiver. A blood glucose calibration is when the child checks their blood glucose level using a finger poke and enters the information into the receiver. This allows the CGM system to determine whether the blood glucose readings from the sensor are accurate, or whether any adjustments to the readings need to occur. Blood glucose calibrations should be done when the blood glucose levels are relatively stable and not rapidly changing.

Different CGM systems are available in different countries, and new CGM devices are continually being developed. If you are interested in this technology, you can discuss with your diabetes team which CGM systems are available in your area.

Uses and Advantages of CGM

Some of the potential uses and advantages of using CGM technology include:

- Potentially less finger-poke blood glucose testing
- More blood glucose information to help with insulin dose adjustments
- May reduce number of low blood glucose levels, particularly overnight
- Alarms to detect high and low blood glucose levels
- Potential to combine with insulin pumps to have automatic adjustments to basal insulin rates in response to blood glucose levels
- Information on what direction the blood glucose is predicted to move (often in the next 15 to 30 minutes)

For many children, one of the biggest advantages of CGM is the decrease in blood glucose finger pokes. For parents, especially those of younger children, the biggest advantage of these devices is being able to know what the blood glucose level is during the night without having to wake their child.

CGM technology provides a lot of data and, when used properly, can help with pattern recognition and insulin dose adjustments. Families may identify that their child is having low glucose levels in the night, for example, which they hadn't detected otherwise. Alarms can be set to alert when the blood glucose is high or low. In addition, the presence of the glucose trend arrows allows for more accurate corrections of high or low blood glucose levels. For example, a high blood glucose reading with an associated trend arrow pointing up (indicating the glucose levels are rising) will need a bigger insulin correction than a high blood glucose reading with an associated trend arrow going down.

Pitfalls and Disadvantages of CGM

Here are some of the potential pitfalls and disadvantages of using CGM technology.

- More blood glucose information may be overwhelming or confusing.
- Having to wear a device on the body all of the time may not be ideal.
- Technical problems related to the delay between sensor and blood glucose readings, or interference from medications (for example, acetaminophen) may occur.

- CGM platforms may be less accurate in the initial period after sensor insertion; this time period varies.
- Skin irritation from the tapes used to secure the CGM may occur.
- Too many alarms for high or low blood glucose levels can interfere with sleep and activities.
- The cost of a CGM device may be quite high and may not be covered by personal health insurance.

While the thought of having more information about glucose readings can initially seem like a good idea, it can be overwhelming. This continuous source of information can make some families and children feel like they can never escape from the diabetes. Reacting right away to "one-off" changes, rather than looking out for consistent blood glucose patterns, may also lead to too frequent changes to insulin pump settings or insulin injection doses.

For some children and teens, one of the biggest barriers to using CGM technology is the idea of having to wear a device all the time. This may particularly be the case for children who are already wearing an insulin pump.

There are some important technical pitfalls to be aware of when using CGM technology. First, there is a delay in what the blood glucose readings are between the interstitial fluid, where the sensor sits, and the bloodstream. It takes time for the changes in glucose to become equilibrated throughout the body. This is one of the reasons why finger-poke blood glucose readings can be different from sensor readings. Because of this, if a very low or high reading is seen on the sensor, it is always important to confirm the result with a finger-poke blood glucose reading. It also takes up to 12 hours for some of the sensors to start accurately measuring blood glucose levels after they have been inserted. Finger-poke blood glucose levels will be required in the intervening time.

Some medications, in particular acetaminophen (for example, Tylenol), can interfere with the sensor and make the blood glucose readings inaccurate for several hours.

While CGM is a great way to collect blood glucose information, if the family does not have a way of reviewing the data and making appropriate insulin dose adjustments, its potential to improve diabetes control is limited. All of the CGM devices have different software programs that allow families and diabetes teams to download the information to review. It is important when using CGM that the family is aware of how to download the device and how to understand the information that is displayed, and that this is done at least once a week. Reviewing these CGM downloads with your diabetes team is an important part of routine diabetes care.

> While the thought of having more information about glucose readings can initially seem like a good idea, it can be overwhelming.

Pro Tip

The tapes used to secure the CGM devices can cause irritation or rashes, particularly in children and teens with more sensitive skin.

Closed Insulin Loops/Artificial Pancreas

One exciting current area of research is in closed-loop insulin systems, otherwise known as the artificial pancreas. This is where a CGM is used along with insulin pump therapy: the sensor tells the insulin pump how much insulin to give throughout the day and night — no information needs to be entered into the pump. Some pump-CGM systems can already do partial automatic adjustments, such as decreasing or turning off the basal insulin if the blood glucose is low. With a completely closed-loop system, there would be adjustments for both low and high blood glucose levels, to try to keep the blood glucose levels in target range for the majority of the day.

Researching the Cause and a Possible Cure

In chapter 1, we explained that diabetes is an autoimmune disorder caused when a genetic predisposition or susceptibility is triggered by something in the environment. Over the past 20 years, there have been enormous advances in our understanding of the genetic aspects of type 1 diabetes, although pieces of the puzzle remain to be found.

The Genetic Link

> Over the past 20 years, there have been enormous advances in our understanding of the genetic aspects of type 1 diabetes.

There are a number of genes involved in making a person susceptible to type 1 diabetes; the most important appears to lie in what is called the **histocompatibility locus antigen** (HLA), or the "tissue-typing" region of chromosome six. This region contains genes that control the body's immune responses — for example, how we deal with foreign materials such as viruses, bacteria and toxins. In people susceptible to diabetes, these genes appear to be somewhat impaired.

Contained in this region of chromosome six are genes that determine different levels of susceptibility or risk of developing type 1 diabetes, while other genes actually allow resistance to diabetes. Could this resistance be harnessed and turned into a therapy that could alter these impaired genes and protect against diabetes? This is an important question, and a good deal of current research is focused on this.

The Environmental Link

In the hunt for environmental triggers that may "wake up" a genetic predisposition to diabetes, there has been extensive research focusing on viruses, food products and environmental toxins. This research has not yielded consistent results, nor has it identified a single trigger for the development of diabetes, but studies are still ongoing.

Researchers hope to identify a viral or other infectious agent responsible for causing the pancreatic damage so they can work on developing a vaccine against it. This could possibly prevent diabetes. Avoiding certain toxins could have a similar effect. There are studies in progress that test these theories in both animals and humans.

Assessing Risk

Once the genes and the environment align themselves in a way that starts the progression toward diabetes, a series of events occur that are now quite well understood and are being studied in greater detail. The immune system and environmental changes lead to an inflammatory response (insulitis) in the islet cells where insulin is made. Antibodies to some of the proteins in the islets appear in the blood. Detecting these antibodies allows us to determine who may be at high risk for developing diabetes.

Most of the studies have been and are being performed on close relatives (parents, children and siblings) of people with diabetes because, as you'd expect in any disorder with a genetic link, the risk to family members is much higher than in the general population. The problem is that diabetes in family members accounts for only 5% to 10% of all new cases of type 1 diabetes. Studies in the general population have been much more difficult to perform and may not be as useful for predictions as those in close relatives.

Preventing the Immune Response

Studies in animals have shown that diabetes can be prevented by exposure to a number of medications that decrease the immune response. These include some medications with serious side effects — such as those used to prevent the rejection of transplanted organs or those used in other autoimmune conditions — as well as much safer agents, such as the vitamin B_3 product nicotinamide and the hormone insulin. Present studies in the United States, Canada, Australia and Europe are evaluating the possibility of preventing diabetes in high-risk groups by giving these types of medications.

Preventing the Progression of Diabetes

For those who already have diabetes, two different lines of research are looking at ways to reverse the condition: immune interventions at diagnosis to stop further damage to the pancreas and maintain the "honeymoon period"; and transplanting the pancreas, or at least the islet cells, to reverse the condition once it is fully established.

So far, interventions at diagnosis have been either unsuccessful or minimally successful, and there are currently no treatments approved for routine use.

Whole-Pancreas Transplants

The first whole-pancreas transplants were attempted in the 1960s, and transplants continue to be performed in many centers around the world. The problem with this operation is that the transplanted pancreas can undergo rejection. People who have a pancreas transplant therefore need high doses of antirejection medications, which can have troublesome and significant side effects, including development of cancer and type 2 diabetes.

For people who need a kidney transplant for advanced diabetes-related kidney complications, and who will need antirejection drugs anyway, transplanting the pancreas at the same time makes good sense. For those well controlled on insulin, with no evidence of kidney complications, transplantation is usually not the best choice.

Islet Cell Transplants

Enormous efforts have been made not only to perfect pancreatic transplantation, but also to isolate the islets (the insulin-producing cells) and transplant them without the non–insulin-producing parts of the pancreas. Recent advances in islet-transplantation technology have improved the outlook for this procedure, but extensive testing is still required before it becomes more common.

People who receive transplanted islet cells still require immunosuppressive drugs thereafter, to prevent rejection of the transplanted cells. Even if the technical and rejection problems can be fixed, it is expected that two to three organ donors' pancreases will be needed for each islet-transplant recipient. This is a major stumbling block to islet-cell transplants becoming a realistic solution to type 1 diabetes.

At this stage, islet cell transplants are mainly performed in adults with poorly controlled type 1 diabetes, and particularly in those adults with frequent and severe low blood glucose episodes.

Pro Tip

Virtually no transplants have been performed in young people with diabetes.

Creating New Islet Cells

The next phase of research involves genetic engineering, in which either animal or non-islet cells are genetically changed to become functioning islet cells. This area of research is often referred to as stem cell therapy.

The enormous complexity of islet cell function is being unraveled steadily. This is helping researchers target the genes that must function to make the cells produce and secrete insulin in response to changes in blood glucose levels.

Although scientists have made significant breakthroughs in being able to produce functioning islet cells, there remain two major areas where further research is needed. The first is that these newly formed islet cells are still at risk of being damaged by the immune reaction (the antibodies) that caused the diabetes to occur in the first place. Technology to develop special capsules to contain the newly formed islet cells and keep them away from the antibodies is ongoing. The second major area of research needed is around making sure that these new islet cells don't change into different types of cells, particularly cancer cells. Major steps have been taken in the past five years to tackle these issues, and the hope is that sometime in the future this therapy may become a realistic treatment option.

> The enormous complexity of islet cell function is being unraveled steadily. This is helping researchers target the genes that must function to make the cells produce and secrete insulin in response to changes in blood glucose levels.

Where Do We Go from Here?

Around the world, many researchers remain focused on questions to do with the causes, course and complications of type 1 and type 2 diabetes. They continue to make steady progress, but for many people, the pace is too slow. It is clear that there is an ever-increasing need for funding to support research and treatment programs.

Children with diabetes, their families and health care providers, and government and nongovernmental organizations that fund diabetes care and research, must focus on the challenge at hand: to provide the best available care for people with the disease. It is easy to become frustrated. Those receiving insulin will always hope that a major advance is just around the corner. We need, however, to balance this hope against the reality of where we are in research and how far we are likely to advance in the next few years.

Following the steps to maintain excellent physical and emotional health now is of critical importance. That way, when something better comes along in terms of a treatment or cure, your children will be well positioned to benefit.

Did You Know?
Cause for Optimism

The history of diabetes since the discovery of insulin in 1921 is one of steady progress in all aspects of this group of disorders: cause, course and complications. More is to be expected, culminating in the development of either a technological or biological artificial pancreas. This day cannot come soon enough.

Q & A

Q. I keep reading about ancient cures for diabetes and alternative nondrug remedies. How do I know what to believe?

A. Children with type 1 diabetes require insulin; unfortunately, there is no therapy, alternative or otherwise, that eliminates that need. Some people with diabetes find that certain nutritional supplements make them feel better. These are probably not harmful, but shouldn't be thought of as part of the diabetes routine. Check with your diabetes team before taking them.

Some people with diabetes find that certain nutritional supplements make them feel better.

Q. We are a family of five. One of our children has diabetes. How can the rest of us find out if we are at high risk for developing diabetes, and be part of a prevention study?

A. The best way to learn about important clinical research and how you can be involved is to talk to your diabetes team. If your child is not receiving ongoing care from a pediatric diabetes team and your doctor is unaware of research opportunities that may interest you, you may want to request referral to a children's center.

Pro Tip

Join the American Diabetes Association or Diabetes Canada, as well as the Juvenile Diabetes Research Foundation. Membership in these organizations includes a subscription to their publications, which always feature the latest research.

Q. Every week, I read a story in the paper about some new treatment for diabetes being just around the corner. Yet I have had diabetes for 25 years and my child has had it for six years. We both need to take insulin injections, do blood glucose checking and continue to worry about control. Why do the media report premature research findings?

A. It's true that a "cure" always seems to be around the corner. There are many reasons why stories often promise more than they deliver. Sometimes, the media misinterpret or sensationalize the information they receive from medical meetings or medical journals. Other times, the researchers themselves give an overly optimistic view of when their research will "bear fruit" and change diabetes care. Still other times, research that looks promising in its early stages turns out to be not as exciting as the studies continue. Unexpected problems may emerge as treatments are studied over the long haul; initially promising results may not hold up. Read media reports carefully, and ask your health care team or diabetes association about them.

> There are many reasons why stories often promise more than they deliver.

Q. How can I make sure that I hear about the latest important research in diabetes?

A. Look to your diabetes team to keep you informed about research that will make a difference to you or your child. It is their responsibility to stay up-to-date on current treatments and significant advances. You may also find useful information on the internet (see Further Resources, at the end of this book).

Afterword

Let us **reinforce** a few key messages:

Key Messages

- Type 1 diabetes is a serious condition, with significant short- and long-term consequences.

- The better the overall blood glucose control, the better the long-term outcome.

- Achieving the goals of treatment can be difficult work.

- Behavior around diabetes routines is key to good blood glucose control and positive outcomes.

- We're in this together — teamwork!

We end this book with a few thoughts.

History Recap

The discovery of insulin remains one of the 20th century's greatest medical advances, transforming a previously uniformly fatal disease into a chronic disorder with serious consequences.

The story of type 1 diabetes really begins with the isolation of insulin by the University of Toronto researchers — led by Frederick Banting; his science student Charles Best; J.J.R. Macleod, the professor of physiology who provided lab facilities and support; and J.B. Collip, the Albertan biochemist. Truth be told, other researchers were hot on their heels, but they were first. The discovery of insulin remains one of the 20th century's greatest medical advances, transforming a previously uniformly fatal disease into a chronic condition with serious consequences.

Insulin has garnered three Nobel Prizes: in 1923 to Banting and Macleod for its discovery; in 1958 to Frederick Sanger for elucidating its biochemical structure; and in 1977 to Rosalyn Yalow for developing methods to measure insulin levels in the body (her research partner Solomon Berson had died and, therefore, was not eligible to be named on the prize).

The parallel story is about those individuals who were fading away as a result of their diabetes when this miraculous new agent became available. Leonard Thompson, then 14 years of age, was the first to receive insulin, at Toronto General Hospital. His chart, now on display, shows a physician's order to administer "7.5 cc of Macleod's serum in each buttock." Thompson was followed in rapid succession by others such as Teddy Rider and Elizabeth Hughes, who wrote to her parents in the United States about the "unspeakably wonderful" effects of this new medication.

Subsequent Advances in Diabetes Care

- Insulin preparations have led the way: first, with the development of methods of purifying insulin from beef then pork pancreases; then with manipulation of this short-acting insulin (originally called regular insulin) to produce longer- or intermediate-acting insulins NPH and Lente; next was the use of recombinant DNA technology to produce human insulin biosynthetically, quickly ending the use of animal-derived preparations almost completely; and finally to preparations of insulins biosynthetically tailored to be very short- or long-acting (insulin analogs) — including insulin lispro, aspart and others in the fast-acting category, and insulin glargine and detemir in the long-acting group. Next steps will likely include very, very long-acting background or basal insulin that is given, for example, once a week or once a month.

- The monitoring of glucose control started with detection of glucose in the urine: if the urine was negative for glucose, the preceding blood glucose was presumed to be below about 145 to 180 mg/dL (8 to 10 mmol/L), the level at which, on average, glucose begins to spill into the urine from the blood. Starting in the late 1970s, urine testing was replaced with blood glucose testing techniques. At that time, a senior diabetes physician predicted that "children would *never* take to pricking their fingers repeatedly." Within six months of this prediction, blood glucose monitoring had replaced urine testing. This remains the most expensive aspect of the diabetes treatment routine.

- Technological advances were bound to impact diabetes care in a profound manner: first, with advanced insulins and better monitoring equipment, then with insulin pumps, and more recently with continuous blood glucose sensors. The artificial pancreas is the next big step — that is, a pump that both senses blood glucose level and responds to it by increasing or decreasing infusion of insulin. Prototypes are currently in advanced stages of development. Following that, we hope to see an implantable device that delivers insulin into the liver (via a vein called the portal vein) to best mimic how the nondiabetic pancreas responds.

- While technology to control blood glucose levels has advanced incredibly in the past 30 to 40 years, we still seem to be a long way from preventing diabetes from happening in the first place or reversing it once it has been diagnosed. One can only hope for the development of newer technologies that can solve these issues.

Final Thoughts

At this point in time, there are really no careers that remain closed to people with diabetes.

One of the great joys in having been involved in the lives of so many children and teens with type 1 diabetes and their families is running into them or their parents many years after they have transitioned to an adult center. The young people are often unrecognizable as mature adults; their parents are almost always the key to remembering them. A couple have gone on to become pediatric or adult endocrinologists and certified diabetes educators, while others span the full range of careers. At this point in time, there are really no careers that remain closed to people with diabetes. Inevitably, most will say that our diabetes team helped them stay on the right track. Some will say a simple thank you.

Each of us goes into a field of work for very personal reasons. For one of us (Denis Daneman), the choice of diabetes care was greatly influenced by the presence of strong role models while at medical school, but also significantly so by a strong family history in his wife's family: first, her maternal grandfather developed diabetes in 1928 and had to wait six months before insulin became available. He lived until age 94, having had diabetes for more than 60 years. His secret to longevity: a strong family history of longevity, plus careful attention to what he ate and a commitment to exercise. By the time of his death, he had received well over 40,000 insulin injections, according to Dr. Daneman's calculations. His grandson — Dr. Daneman's brother-in-law — has had diabetes for almost 50 years and follows his grandfather's example when it comes to food and exercise. This personal story is presented to demonstrate the benefits of good self-care.

We hope this book has been worth your while.

Note from a "Graduate"

One of us recently received this note:

You may not remember me. I was diagnosed with type 1 diabetes at the age of 2. You were my doctor for many years until I was too old to keep coming to the children's hospital. I just wanted to reach out to say that without your team's guidance and knowledge to share with my parents that I probably wouldn't have grown up a healthy human being. So I want to thank you for taking care of me and helping control my diabetes. I am always working to control it better every day. It is a struggle at times, but that comes with it, I suppose. At 33 years of age, I am healthy with no complications of the diabetes. I live a healthy lifestyle and again it all began with you. So thank you again for all your time and knowledge.

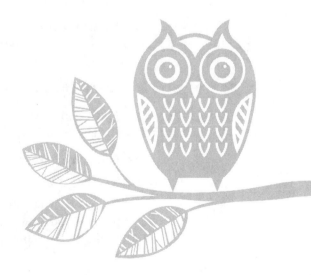

Glossary

A1c: *see* Hemoglobin A1c test.

Albuminuria: presence of protein in the urine. In small amounts, called microalbuminuria, this signals early diabetic nephropathy. Larger amounts, called overt proteinuria or macroproteinuria, suggests advanced nephropathy.

Angiotensin converting enzyme (ACE) inhibitors: medications used to protect the kidney once early nephropathy or high blood pressure has been detected.

Antibodies: proteins produced by the immune system to neutralize foreign proteins (i.e., infectious agents).

Autoimmune disorder: a disease in which the body's immune system mistakenly attacks the body's own tissues. Type 1 diabetes is the result of an autoimmune disorder.

Basal insulin: the background insulin required to manage blood glucose during sleep and during periods of fasting throughout the day.

Beta cells: cells in the islets of Langerhans in the pancreas that produce insulin.

Body mass index (BMI): an indicator of the child's size, with weight corrected for height.

Bolus insulin: short- or fast-acting insulin that is given with carbohydrate-containing meals and snacks or used to correct blood glucose levels that are higher than target.

CGMS: continuous glucose monitoring system.

CSII: continuous subcutaneous insulin infusion (also called pump therapy).

Carbohydrate: a major source of energy for the body (sugar and starches).

Correction factor: refers to the units of insulin required to correct an out-of-target blood glucose so that it returns to the desired range.

Diabetic ketoacidosis (DKA): severe dehydration and acidosis that develop when blood glucose is very high and not enough insulin is available to prevent excessive breakdown of fat.

DKA: *see* Diabetic ketoacidosis.

Endocrinologist: physician specializing in the diagnosis and treatment of diabetes and other disorders involving the endocrine (glandular) system.

Enuresis: bed-wetting.

Glucagon: hormone produced in the pancreas that increases blood glucose by stimulating the liver to release its glucose stores.

Glucose: the substance required by the cells of the body to supply energy. Sometimes used interchangeably with *sugar*.

Glycogen: substance made up of glucose that is stored in the liver and muscles. When cells require glucose for energy, glycogen is changed back into glucose and released into the blood.

Glycosuria: glucose in the urine.

Gram: unit of weight in the metric system. There are approximately 30 grams in 1 ounce.

Hemoglobin A1c test: blood test used to measure long-term glucose control. Glucose attaches to the hemoglobin in red blood cells in proportion to the average blood glucose level over the life span of the red blood cell (about three months). Measuring A1c levels every three months is the best way to track long-term glucose control.

Histocompatibility locus antigens (HLA): "tissue-typing" genes on chromosome six that can control the body's immune response and provide information on someone's risk of developing diabetes.

Hyperglycemia: blood glucose levels above the range seen in those without diabetes.

Hyperlipidemia: blood fat levels (cholesterol and triglycerides) above the normal range for age and sex.

Hypoglycemia: blood glucose levels below the range seen in those without diabetes.

Hypoglycemic reaction: symptoms associated with a lower-than-normal blood glucose level.

Immune system: a complex system that defends the body against viruses, bacteria and other invaders. Sometimes the system malfunctions; *see* Autoimmune disorder.

Insulin: hormone produced in the pancreas that is essential for normal metabolism of glucose.

Insulin analog: insulin biologically altered to change its onset, peak and duration of action.

Insulin-to-carbohydrate ratio: the amount of carbohydrate, measured in grams, that 1 unit of insulin metabolizes. This ratio varies from one person to the next and may even vary throughout the day for any one person.

Islet cell antibodies: antibodies to proteins in the pancreas, often found at the time of diagnosis (or even before diagnosis) of diabetes. Used to detect those at risk of diabetes.

Islets of Langerhans: small clusters of cells within the pancreas responsible for the secretion of insulin and other pancreatic hormones.

Ketoacidosis: *see* Diabetic ketoacidosis.

Ketones: breakdown products of fat metabolism, which contribute to development of DKA.

Lipids: fats.

Lipoatrophy: disappearance of fatty tissue at the injection sites.

Lipohypertrophy: accumulation of fat at injection sites.

Macrovascular complications: diabetes-related complications that affect the large blood vessels, causing heart attacks, strokes and poor circulation to the extremities, most commonly the feet.

Macula: area near the center of the eye's retina, responsible for precise vision.

Microalbuminuria: *see* Albuminuria.

Microvascular complications: diabetes-related complications that affect the small blood vessels, such as nephropathy, neuropathy and retinopathy.

Nephropathy: kidney damage that may occur as a result of diabetes.

Neuroglycopenia: deficiency in glucose supply to the brain.

Neuropathy: nerve damage that may occur as a result of diabetes.

Nocturia: urination at night.

Ophthalmologist: physician who specializes in the diagnosis and treatment of diseases of the eye.

Overt proteinuria: *see* Albuminuria.

Pancreas: organ in the abdomen, behind the stomach, that produces both digestive juices and hormones such as insulin and glucagon.

Pediatric endocrinologist: a pediatrician who specializes in disorders of the endocrine (hormonal) system.

Pediatrician: doctor specializing in the care of health problems in children and teens.

Polydipsia: excessive fluid drinking.

Polyphagia: excessive food intake.

Polyuria: excessive urination.

Retina: center part of the back lining of the eye, which senses light. Its many small blood vessels may become damaged when someone has diabetes for a long time.

Retinopathy: eye damage that may occur as a result of diabetes.

Target range: range of blood glucose within which most results of blood glucose testing should fall.

Thyroid: gland in the lower neck that makes thyroid hormones.

Type 1 diabetes: a form of diabetes that usually begins in childhood and requires treatment with insulin.

Type 2 diabetes: a form of diabetes that usually develops as people age and can usually be managed through changes in diet and lifestyle.

Further Resources

Organizations

Juvenile Diabetes Research Foundation (JDRF)

JDRF is the leading global organization focused on type 1 diabetes research. The goal of JDRF research is to improve the lives of all people affected by type 1 diabetes by accelerating progress on the most promising opportunities for curing, better treating and preventing type 1 diabetes.

Phone: 1-800-533-CURE (2873)
Email: info@jdrf.org
International website: www.jdrf.org
Canadian website: www.jdrf.ca
For the newly diagnosed: www.jdrf.ca/living-with-t1d/newly-diagnosed

American Diabetes Association (ADA)

The American Diabetes Association is a United States–based association working to fight the consequences of diabetes and to help those affected by diabetes.

Phone: 1-800-DIABETES (342-2383)
Email: askADA@diabetes.org
Website: www.diabetes.org

Diabetes Canada (DC)
(previously the Canadian Diabetes Association)

Diabetes Canada is a registered national charity whose mission includes serving the 11 million Canadians living with diabetes or prediabetes.

Phone: 1-800-BANTING (226-8464)
Email: info@diabetes.ca
Website: www.diabetes.ca

International Society for Pediatric and Adolescent Diabetes (ISPAD)

ISPAD is the only international society focusing on all types of diabetes in the worldwide population under the age of 25.

Phone: +49 (0)30 24603-210
Email: secretariat@ispad.org
Website: www.ispad.org

> **Note:** There are differences in some of the recommendations made in the three major guidelines on page 226 (ADA, DC and ISPAD). We regard these as relatively minor and feel that the differences arise from subtle differences in interpretation of the available facts. These differences ought not cause confusion in the treatment of a child or teen with type 1 or type 2 diabetes.

Children with Diabetes
Informational website.
Website: www.childrenwithdiabetes.com

Clinical Practice and Diabetes Management Guidelines

American Diabetes Association

American Diabetes Association 2016 Guidelines: www.ndei.org/ADA-diabetes-management-guidelines-diagnosis-A1C-testing.aspx.html.

"Standards of Medical Care in Diabetes – 2018." *Diabetes Care.* 2018; 41 (Supplement 1): S1–2: http://care.diabetesjournals.org/content/41/Supplement_1/S1.

"Children and Adolescents: Standards of Medical Care in Diabetes — 2018." *Diabetes Care.* 2018 Jan; 41 (Supplement 1): S126–36.

Diabetes Canada

Clinical Practice Guidelines 2018: http://guidelines.diabetes.ca.

Full reference guide: *Canadian Journal of Diabetes.* 2013 Apr (Supplement 1): 37: http://guidelines.diabetes.ca/app_themes/cdacpg/resources/cpg_2013_full_en.pdf.

2018 Clinical Practice Guidelines, Quick Reference Guide: http://guidelines.diabetes.ca/docs/CPG-quick-reference-guide-web-EN.pdf.

International Society for Pediatric and Adolescent Diabetes

ISPAD Clinical Practice Consensus Guidelines 2014: www.ispad.org/default.asp?page=ISPADClinicalPract.

Topic-Specific Resources

Driving and Diabetes

American Diabetes Association
"Diabetes and Driving": https://doi.org/10.2337/dc12-s081.

Diabetes Canada
"Guidelines for Diabetes and Private and Commercial Driving": www.diabetes.ca/diabetes-and-you/healthy-living-resources/ general-tips/guidelines-for-diabetes-and-private-and-commercial.

Exercise and Diabetes

American Diabetes Association
Colberg S.R., Sigal R.J., Yardley J.E., et al. "Physical Activity/ Exercise and Diabetes: A Position Statement of the American Diabetes Association." *Diabetes Care*. 2016 Nov; 39 (11): 2065–79: http://dx.doi.org/10.2337/dc16-1728.

Diabetes Canada
"Physical Activity & Exercise": www.diabetes.ca/clinical-practice-education/professional-resources/physical-activity-exercise.

International Society for Pediatric and Adolescent Diabetes
Robertson K., Riddell M.C., Guinhouya B.C., et al. "ISPAD Clinical Practice Consensus Guidelines 2014: Exercise in Children and Adolescents with Diabetes." *Pediatric Diabetes*. 2014 Sep; 15 (Supplement 20): 203–23: www.ispad.org/resource/ resmgr/Docs/CPCG_2014_CHAP_14.pdf.

Nutrition and Diabetes

MyPlate
www.choosemyplate.gov

MyPlate is the United States Department of Agriculture (USDA) Food Guide website. It is a reminder to find your healthy eating style and build it throughout your lifetime. Everything you eat and drink matters. The right mix can help you be healthier now and in the future. This means:

- Focus on variety, amount and nutrition
- Choose foods and beverages with less saturated fat, sodium and added sugars
- Start with small changes to build healthier eating styles
- Support healthy eating for everyone

Canada's Food Guides
www.canada.ca/en/health-canada/services/canada-food-guides.html

Canadian Nutrient File (CNF) — Search by Food
https://food-nutrition.canada.ca/cnf-fce/index-eng.jsp

Glycemic Index
The Glycemic Index (GI) is a relative ranking of carbohydrate
    in foods according to how they affect blood glucose levels:
    www.glycemicindex.com.

School and Diabetes

American Diabetes Association
"Safe at School": www.diabetes.org/living-with-diabetes/parents-
    and-kids/diabetes-care-at-school.

Diabetes Canada
"Kids with Diabetes at School": www.diabetes.ca/kidsatschool.

Diabetes at School
www.diabetesatschool.ca

Canadian Paediatric Society and Diabetes Canada 2017
"Advocacy Tip Sheet: How You Can Advocate for Improved
    Student Support": www.cps.ca/uploads/advocacy/2017-18_
    Diabetes@School_advocacy_tip_sheet.pdf.

Travel and Diabetes

American Diabetes Association
"Air Travel and Diabetes": www.diabetes.org/living-with-diabetes/
    know-your-rights/discrimination/public-accommodations/air-
    travel-and-diabetes.

Beyondtype1.org
"Airport Security": https://beyondtype1.org/airport-security-and-
    type-1-diabetes.

Canadian Air Transport Security Authority
"Diabetic Supplies": www.catsa-acsta.gc.ca/en/item/diabetic-
    supplies.

Using an Insulin Pen

American Diabetes Association
The ADA's *Diabetes Forecast* magazine (www.diabetesforecast.org)
    features a number of useful articles about insulin pens.

The Hospital for Sick Children
"Pens and Cartridges": www.aboutkidshealth.ca/Article?contentid=
    1732&language=English.

Books

Anderson, Karri. *I Have Diabetes: A Children's Book About Juvenile Diabetes*. Createspace Independent Publishing, 2012.

Betschart-Roemer, Jean. *It's Time to Learn about Diabetes: A Workbook on Diabetes for Children*. Hoboken, NJ: Wiley, 1995.

Brackenridge, Betty Page, and Richard R. Rubin. *Sweet Kids: How to Balance Diabetes Control and Good Nutrition with Family Peace*. American Diabetes Association, 1996.

Calentine, Leighann. *Kids First, Diabetes Second: Tips for Parenting a Child with Type 1 Diabetes*. Ann Arbor, MI: Spry Publishing, 2012.

Grunes, Barbara, and Linda R. Yoakam. *Diabetes Snacks, Treats, and Easy Eats for Kids: 150 Recipes for the Foods Kids Really Like to Eat*. Evanston, IL: Agate Surrey, 2017.

Hively, Holly K. *I'm Just Like Everyone Else: A Book about Children Thriving with Type 1 Diabetes*. Createspace Independent Publishing, 2017.

Kaufman, Miriam. *Easy for You to Say. Q and As for Teens Living with Chronic Illness or Disabilities*. Toronto: Firefly Books, 2005.

Laffel, Lori M.B., Deborah A. Butler, Laurie A. Higgins, Margaret T. Lawlor, and Cynthia A. Pasquarello. *Joslin's Guide to Managing Childhood Diabetes — A Family Teamwork Approach*. Boston: Joslin Diabetes Center, 2001.

McCarthy, Moira and Jake Kushner. *Raising Teens with Diabetes: A Survival Guide for Parents*. Ann Arbor, MI: Spry Publishing, 2013.

Riddell, Michael. *Getting Pumped! An Insulin Pump Guide for Active Individuals with Type 1 Diabetes*. www.getting pumped.org.

Wysocki, Tim. *The Ten Keys to Helping Your Child Grow Up with Diabetes*. American Diabetes Association, 2004.

Articles of Note

American Diabetes Association. "Children and Adolescents." *Diabetes Care*. 2017 Jan; 40 (Supplement 1): S105–13.

Riddell M.C., Gallen I.W., Smart C.E., et al. "Exercise Management in Type 1 Diabetes: A Consensus Statement." *Lancet: Diabetes Endocrinology*. 2017 May; 5 (5): 377–90.

Library and Archives Canada Cataloguing in Publication

Daneman, Denis, author
    When a child has diabetes / Denis Daneman, MBBCh, FRCPC,
Shaun Barrett, RN, MN, CDE, Jennifer Harrington, MD, PhD, FRACP. — 4th edition.

Includes index.
ISBN 978-0-7788-0613-4 (softcover)

    1. Diabetes in children—Popular works. I. Barrett, Shaun, author
II. Harrington, Jennifer, 1977-, author III. Title.

RJ420.D5D36 2018   618.92'462   C2018-902985-4

Index

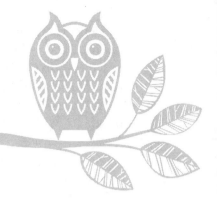

cough syrup, 87
CSII (continuous subcutaneous insulin infusions). *See* insulin pumps
cyclamate, 115

D

day camps, 167–68
dehydration, 16, 83, 92
depression, 21
detemir, 48
dextrose. *See* sugars, fast-acting
diabetes mellitus, 10–25. *See also* complications; diabetes, type 1; diabetes, type 2
  diagnosing, 13
  financial concerns, 103, 138
  risk factors, 91
  types, 13–14
diabetes, type 1, 225
  adjusting to, 122–27
  advances in care, 207–12, 219–20
  alternative remedies, 216
  associated conditions, 182–83
  causes, 14–15
  complications, 18, 128–29
  diagnosing, 15, 16
  emotional reactions to, 20–22, 25, 116–19
  and employment, 158
  family issues, 119–20, 126
  helpful hints, 158–59
  honeymoon period (remission), 17, 24–25
  in the long term, 18–20, 116–40, 219
  onset, 16–17
  and pregnancy, 155
  preventing progression, 214–15
  psychosocial factors, 118, 127

  research into, 19, 36, 134, 195, 206–7, 212–15
  risk factors, 24, 213, 216
  self-management of, 131–32
  stages, 16–20
  tasks involved, 26–33
  telling friends about, 120–21
  therapies for, 206–17
diabetes, type 2, 89–97, 225
  asymptomatic, 91
  causes, 15, 90–91
  complications, 96–97, 196
  incidence, 89–90
  managing, 93–96
  medications for, 94–96, 97
  preventing, 97
  symptoms, 91–92
diabetes burnout, 125, 133–34
diabetes team, 25, 27, 179–81
  teenagers and, 151, 152
diabetic ketoacidosis (DKA), 17, 18, 80–82, 223
  cause, 87
  symptoms, 81, 88
  in type 2 diabetes, 92
diets (weight-loss), 94
drinks, 104. *See also* alcohol
driving, 157
drugs (recreational), 154–55

E

eating disorders, 155–56
eating out, 113
emergency preparedness, 174
employment, 158
endocrinologists, 22, 179, 223. *See also* diabetes team
enuresis, 16
environment, 15, 212–13
estrogen, 40
exercise. *See* physical activity

eye problems, 18, 197, 198, 204, 225

F

families, 119–20, 126, 180–81.
    See also parents
family doctors, 184, 191
fasting, 114
fatigue, 16
fats, 11, 103
fiber, 102
field trips, 147, 166–67
flu shots, 44, 204
food, 98–115. *See also* meal
    planning
    appetite for, 107, 145
    and blood glucose levels, 37–39,
        100–104
    "free," 104
    gluten-containing, 203
    glycemic index of, 111–13
    in healthy diet, 93–94
    insulin and, 11–12, 108
    intake adjustments, 65, 171–72
    for sick days, 84
    timing of, 27, 51
food guides, 99
foot problems, 201, 204

G

genetics, 14, 212
gestational diabetes, 13
glargine, 48
glucagon, 11, 40, 75–79, 223
    emergency use, 76, 166
    mini-dose, 78–79
Glucophage, 94–95
glucose, 11–12. *See also* blood
    glucose levels
glulisine, 48

gluten intolerance, 182–83, 197,
    203
glycemic index, 111–13
glycogen, 12, 223
glycosuria, 16, 223
goiter, 182
Graves' disease, 202
grief, 20
growth, 39–40

H

Hashimoto's thyroiditis, 182,
    197, 202
health insurance, 55
hemoglobin A1c, 18–20, 150,
    223
high blood pressure
    (hypertension), 196, 197
HLA (histocompatibility locus
    antigen), 212, 223
hormones. *See specific hormones*
Humalog, 48
Humulin-N, 47, 48
hunger, 107, 145
hyperglycemia (high blood
    glucose), 79–80, 87, 223.
    See also blood glucose levels
    symptoms, 38, 80, 165
hyperlipidemia, 196, 197, 223
hypertension (high blood
    pressure), 196, 197
hyperthyroidism, 202
hypoglycemia (low blood glucose),
    18, 31–32, 69–79, 223.
    See also blood glucose levels
    causes, 70
    mild, 71, 88
    responding to, 31, 72–73,
        75–79, 166
    risk of, 17, 74, 172
    severe, 75–79, 86

islets of Langerhans, 11, 222, 224. *See also* beta cells; pancreas increasing, 214, 215
isophane, 48

K

ketones, 29, 224. *See also* diabetic ketoacidosis
kidney disease (nephropathy), 18, 197, 198–200, 224
kidney infections, 205

L

Lantus, 47, 48
Levemir, 47, 48
lipids. *See* cholesterol; fats
lipoatrophy, 181, 224
lipohypertrophy, 31, 181, 224
lispro, 48

M

macronutrients, 99. *See also* *specific nutrients*
macrovascular complications, 18, 128
macula. *See* retinopathy
marijuana, 154–55
meal planning, 37, 107–11. *See also* food
  children and, 110
  glycemic index and, 112–13
mealtimes, 109, 137
medical-alert bracelets, 31, 33, 88
medications
  and blood glucose, 87
  as diabetes cause, 13, 91
  for type 2 diabetes, 94–96, 97
menstruation, 160
mental health issues, 183

anxiety, 138, 184
depression, 21
metabolic memory, 194
metformin, 94–95
microalbuminuria, 199, 224
micronutrients, 100
microvascular complications, 18, 128
monogenic diabetes, 14

N

neonatal diabetes, 14
nephropathy (kidney disease), 18, 197, 198–200, 224
neuroglycopenia, 71, 225
neuropathy (nerve problems), 18, 197, 200–201, 225
nicotinamide, 213
nocturia, 16, 225
nonalcoholic fatty liver disease (NAFLD), 91, 97
Novolin NPH, 47, 48
NovoRapid, 48
nutrients, 11, 99. *See also* *specific nutrients*
nutrition labels, 105–6
nutrition scales, 106

O

overweight, 15, 91, 196

P

pancreas, 11, 225. *See also* islets of Langerhans
artificial, 212, 219–20
transplants of, 214
parents. *See also* families
  alternate caregivers, 66, 140, 169
  boundary-setting by, 136–37